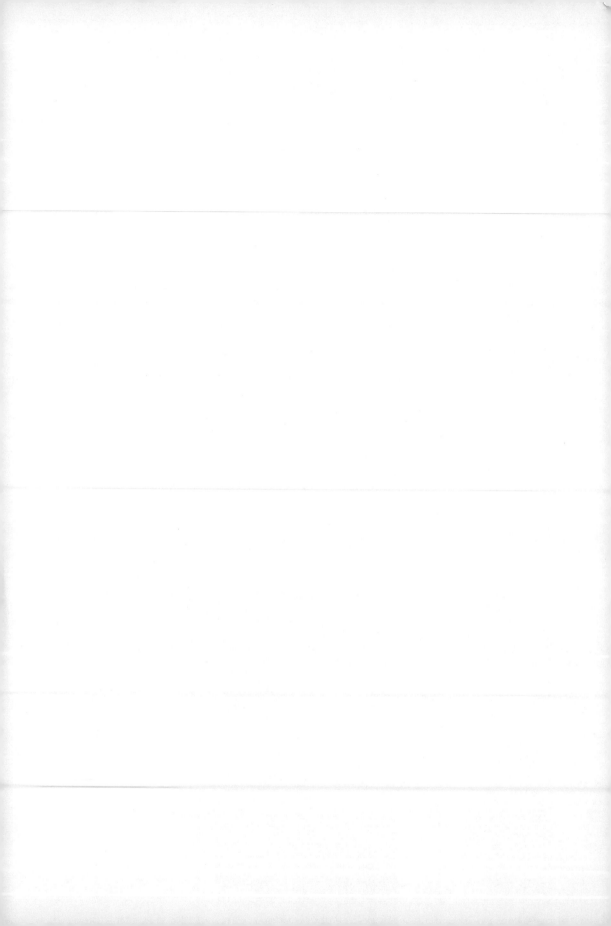

Hyperhidrosis

Editor

DAVID M. PARISER

DERMATOLOGIC CLINICS

www.derm.theclinics.com

Consulting Editor
BRUCE H. THIERS

October 2014 • Volume 32 • Number 4

ELSEVIER

1600 John F. Kennedy Boulevard • Suite 1800 • Philadelphia, Pennsylvania, 19103-2899

http://www.theclinics.com

DERMATOLOGIC CLINICS Volume 32, Number 4
October 2014 ISSN 0733-8635, ISBN-13: 978-0-323-32607-0

Editor: Joanne Husovski
Developmental Editor: Susan Showalter

Dermatologic Clinics (ISSN 0733-8635) is published quarterly by Elsevier Inc., 360 Park Avenue South, New York, NY 10010-1710. Months of publication are January, April, July, and October. Business and editorial offices: 1600 John F. Kennedy Blvd., Suite 1800, Philadelphia, PA 19103-2899. Customer service office: 11830 Westline Drive, St. Louis, MO 63146. Periodicals postage paid at New York, NY, and additional mailing offices. Subscription prices are USD 365.00 per year for US individuals, USD 559.00 per year for US institutions, USD 425.00 per year for Canadian individuals, USD 681.00 per year for Canadian institutions, USD 495.00 per year for international individuals, USD 681.00 per year for international institutions, USD 165.00 per year for US students/residents, and USD 240.00 per year for Canadian and international students/residents. International air speed delivery is included in all *Clinics* subscription prices. All prices are subject to change without notice. **POSTMASTER:** Send address changes to *Dermatologic Clinics*, Elsevier Health Sciences Division, Subscription Customer Service, 3251 Riverport Lane, Maryland Heights, MO 63043. **Customer Service: 1-800-654-2452 (U.S. and Canada); 314-447-8871 (outside U.S. and Canada). Fax: 314-447-8029. E-mail: journalscustomerservice-usa@elsevier.com (for print support); journalsonlinesupport-usa@elsevier.com (for online support).**

Reprints. For copies of 100 or more, of articles in this publication, please contact the Commercial Reprints Department, Elsevier Inc., 360 Park Avenue South, New York, New York 10010-1710. Tel.: 212-633-3874; Fax: 212-633-3820; Email: repritns@elsevier.com.

The *Dermatologic Clinics* is covered in *MEDLINE/PubMed (Index Medicus)*, *Current Contents/Clinical Medicine*, *Excerpta Medica*, *Chemical Abstracts*, and *ISI/BIOMED*.

Contributors

CONSULTING EDITOR

BRUCE H. THIERS, MD
Professor and Chairman, Department of
Dermatology and Dermatologic Surgery,
Medical University of South Carolina,
Charleston, South Carolina

EDITOR

DAVID M. PARISER, MD, FACP, FAAD
Secretary and Founding President,
International Hyperhidrosis Society,
Quakertown, Pennsylvania; Professor,
Department of Dermatology, Eastern
Virginia Medical School, Norfolk, Virginia

AUTHORS

ANGELA BALLARD, RN
International Hyperhidrosis Society,
Quakertown, Pennsylvania

BENJAMIN R. BOHATY, MD
Fellow, Department of Dermatology, The
University of Texas Health Science Center at
Houston, Houston, Texas

TIMUR A. GALPERIN, DO
Clinical Research Fellow, Department of
Dermatology, Saint Louis University School of
Medicine, St Louis, Missouri

DEE ANNA GLASER, MD
Professor and Vice Chairman, Department of
Dermatology, Saint Louis University School of
Medicine, St Louis, Missouri

HENNING HAMM, MD
Professor of Dermatology, Department of
Dermatology, Venereology and Allergology,
University Hospital Würzburg, Würzburg,
Germany

ADELAIDE A. HEBERT, MD
Professor, Departments of Dermatology and
Pediatrics, The University of Texas Health
Science Center at Houston, Houston, Texas

SAMANTHA HILL, MD, FAAD
RidgeView Dermatology, Lynchburg,
Virginia

SUELEN MONTAGNER, MD
Dermatologist Physician, Campinas,
São Paulo, Brazil

ELENI MORAITES, MD
Transitional Resident, Hennepin County
Medical Center, Minneapolis, Minnesota

CHRISTIAN MURRAY, MD, FRCPC
Division of Dermatology, Women's College
Hospital, University of Toronto, Toronto,
Ontario, Canada

DAVID M. PARISER, MD, FACP, FAAD
Secretary and Founding Member, International
Hyperhidrosis Society, Quakertown,
Pennsylvania; Professor, Department of
Dermatology, Eastern Virginia Medical School,
Norfolk, Virginia

LISA J. PIERETTI, MBA
Executive Director and Founding Member,
International Hyperhidrosis Society,
Quakertown, Pennsylvania

NOWELL SOLISH, MD, FRCPC
Division of Dermatology, Women's College
Hospital, University of Toronto, Toronto,
Ontario, Canada

ADA REGINA TRINDADE DE ALMEIDA, MD
Dermatologist Physician, Assistant Physician,
Department of Dermatology, Hospital do
Servidor Público Municipal de São Paulo (SP),
São Paulo, São Paulo, Brazil

OLUSHOLA AKINSHEMOYIN VAUGHN, BA
Student, School of Medicine and Public Health,
University of Wisconsin-Madison, Madison,
Wisconsin

TESSA WEINBERG
School of Medicine, Royal College of Surgeons
of Ireland, Dublin 2, Ireland

Contents

Hyperhidrosis is a skin disorder characterized by excessive sweating that often causes significant impairment in social, occupational, and emotional wellbeing. Hyperhidrosis is thought to affect 2.8% of the US population and can be of primary or secondary origin. Primary hyperhidrosis is usually bilateral, symmetric, and focal. The most common focal sites include, but are not limited to, the palms, soles, and axillae. Secondary hyperhidrosis is usually caused by an underlying medical condition or medication. Secondary hyperhidrosis must be ruled out before a diagnosis of primary hyperhidrosis is made.

Hyperhidrosis is an embarrassing condition that may interfere with routine activities, cause emotional distress, and disturb both professional and social lives of patients. Objective examination is variable and unreliable, so efforts have been made in the last 15 years to substantiate the limitations of these patients, especially in primary focal hyperhidrosis. Almost all therapeutic studies use standardized or self-designed instruments to evaluate the impact of the disease on quality of life and the improvement achieved by treatment. This article gives an overview of the difficulties with which patients with hyperhidrosis are confronted and of research investigating the restrictions.

Hyperhidrosis, characterized by excess sweat production, affects children and adults. Primary focal hyperhidrosis affects any anatomic region with sweat appendages present. Primary hyperhidrosis has traditionally been considered a problem for adults, but approximately 1.6% of adolescents and 0.6% of prepubertal children are affected. Psychological and social development and well-being are often affected, leading to profound emotional and social distress. Quality of life can be improved by early diagnosis and therapy; however, underdiagnosis and lack of knowledge regarding therapeutic options has hindered optimization of therapy in the pediatric population. This article reviews the treatment options for hyperhidrosis with a focus on the pediatric population.

Primary focal hyperhidrosis affects 3% of the US population; about the same number as psoriasis. More than half of these patients have primary focal axillary hyperhidrosis: sweating that is beyond what is anticipated or necessary for thermoregulation.

Most topical therapies are based on aluminum salts, which work by a chemical reaction that forms plugs in the eccrine sweat ducts. Topical anticholinergics may also be used. Instruction on proper methods and timing of antiperspirants enhances effect and may be effective alone or in combination with other treatments in patients with hyperhidrosis.

Iontophoresis is a safe, efficacious, and cost-effective primary treatment of palmar and plantar hyperhidrosis. Decades of clinical experience and research show significant reduction in palmoplantar excessive sweating with minimal side effects. To get the best results from iontophoresis, health care professionals need to provide education on the mechanism of action and benefits, evidence of its use, and creation of a future patient-specific plan of care for continued treatments at home or in the physician's office. Iontophoresis may be combined with other hyperhidrosis treatments, such as topical antiperspirants and botulinum toxin injections.

Botulinum toxin is a safe and effective treatment option for axillary hyperhidrosis. Although its pathophysiology is not clear and somewhat controversial, the beneficial effect of neuromodulators in inhibiting localized sweating temporarily is well known. Before the procedure, correct identification of the affected area is mandatory to avoid wastage of drug and neglect of target areas, and to enhance efficacy, as the hyperhidrotic location may not match the hairy axillary region. Utilization of this medication, such as dilution and injection techniques, depends on medical experience and may have some variations, including methods to make the procedure as painless as possible.

Palmar and plantar hyperhidrosis is relatively common and can have severe psychological and medical consequences for those afflicted. A multitude of treatments exist but are often inadequate especially for those with significant disease. In these cases botulinum neurotoxin provides a reliable method for reducing the symptoms and improving quality of life. Although actual administration is relatively straightforward, pain management is a crucial component that requires a mastery of several techniques. Patients have a high degree of satisfaction with botulinum neurotoxin treatment and are motivated to come back for repeat treatments, usually every 6 months.

Primary hyperhidrosis (HH) commonly affects the axillae, palms, soles, face, and/or the groin. There are limited treatment options available for HH of areas other than the axillae and palms/soles. Botulinum neurotoxin-A is an effective and safe treatment option for most hyperhidrotic areas of the body. Areas that are commonly affected, such as the face and groin, and less common areas like the submammary region and gluteal cleft are discussed. Frey syndrome, compensatory sweating, and postamputation stump HH are also discussed.

Primary hyperhidrosis commonly affects the axillae, palms, soles, scalp, face, and groin. Patients may have multiple areas involved making localized therapy challenging. Systemic therapy may be necessary and can be used as monotherapy or combined with other hyperhidrosis treatments for optimal outcomes. Systemic therapy can also be used to treat secondary hyperhidrosis and compensatory hyperhidrosis.

When medical options for axillary hyperhidrosis have failed, botulinum toxin is an effective, safe, and well-tolerated, although temporary, treatment option. For long-lasting or permanent efficacy, some patients turn to local procedures, such as superficial liposuction or manual curettage, or more invasive local surgery. Newer, minimally invasive treatments have become available, such as microwave energy thermolysis.

Endoscopic thoracic sympathectomy is a surgical technique most commonly used in the treatment of severe palmar hyperhidrosis in selected patients. The procedure also has limited use in the treatment axillary and craniofacial hyperhidrosis. Endoscopic thoracic sympathectomy is associated with a high rate of the development of compensatory hyperhidrosis, which may affect patient satisfaction with the procedure and quality of life.

New therapies are being investigated to treat hyperhidrosis. Novel methods of delivering botulinum toxins and new topical therapies have been developed. Devices that can deliver heat to the area of the eccrine units can reduce sweating. Further studies need to be performed.

The excessive sweating of hyperhidrosis creates profound psychosocial, professional, and financial burdens on the individual sufferer; it contributes to impaired self-worth and self-efficacy, decreased satisfaction in all relationships, avoidance of specific careers, and increased expenditures on everything from clothing to medical treatment. Despite morbidity equal to other well-known dermatologic conditions, hyperhidrosis has historically been underacknowledged and undertreated because of the lack of accessible, scientifically accurate information and dispersal of that information within patient and medical communities. Thankfully, the development of the Internet and the work of the not-for-profit International Hyperhidrosis Society (IHHS) have increased awareness of hyperhidrosis.

Proper billing and coding are essential to document the diagnosis of hyperhidrosis and to assure proper reimbursement for treatment. Providers should become familiar with the payment policies of local health plans to streamline the preauthorization process that is often needed for many treatments commonly used for hyperhidrosis. Having a preprinted letter of medical necessity and patient intake forms that record the necessary historical information about the disease, previous treatments, and other pertinent information will help increase the speed of the office flow. This article presents algorithms for treatment of the various forms of primary focal hyperhidrosis.

DERMATOLOGIC CLINICS

Preface
Hyperhidrosis

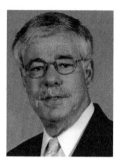

David M. Pariser, MD, FACP, FAAD
Editor

Hyperhidrosis (excessive sweating) is a common condition rarely due to significant underlying pathology that often has serious social, emotional, and professional consequences. It affects about 3% of the population and negatively affects the quality of life of sufferers more than any other disorder that dermatologists treat, as measured by the Dermatology Life Quality Index.

It is most commonly a chronic idiopathic (primary) condition; however, secondary medical conditions or medications should be excluded. Idiopathic hyperhidrosis localized to certain areas of the body is called primary focal hyperhidrosis. Primary focal hyperhidrosis usually affects the axillae, palms, and soles, but other areas such as face and scalp, inframammary area, and groin may also be affected.

This issue is devoted to the diagnosis and treatment of primary focal hyperhidrosis with emphasis on how the disorder affects quality of life. All current treatments are reviewed with an eye to the practical nature of these modalities for the practicing clinician.

After an introduction regarding the incidence, prevalence, and impact on quality of life, there are articles on topical therapies, iontophoresis, and botulinum toxin with attention not only to axillary disease but also other body areas where

it may be used effectively as well. Systemic as well as procedural therapies and surgery as well as emerging and investigational treatments are also discussed. Finally, the practical aspects of incorporating diagnosis and treatment of hyperhidrosis into clinical practice and resources for patients and physicians conclude the issue.

On behalf of the international group of authors, all known for their expertise in hyperhidrosis, I hope that the information presented in this issue will heighten your awareness of this socially disabling problem and that you will appreciate that diagnosis and treatment of patients with primary focal hyperhidrosis is easily learned, leads to a great improvement of patients' quality of life, can be easily integrated into routine office practice, and is economically viable for a busy outpatient practice.

David M. Pariser, MD, FACP, FAAD
Department of Dermatology
Eastern Virginia Medical School
601 Medical Tower
Norfolk, VA 23507, USA

E-mail address:
dpariser@pariserderm.com

Dermatol Clin 32 (2014) xi
http://dx.doi.org/10.1016/j.det.2014.07.001
0733-8635/14/$ – see front matter

Incidence and Prevalence of Hyperhidrosis

Eleni Moraites, MD[a], Olushola Akinshemoyin Vaughn, BA[b], Samantha Hill, MD[c],*

KEYWORDS

- Hyperhidrosis • Primary hyperhidrosis • Secondary hyperhidrosis • Prevalence • Diagnosis

KEY POINTS

- Hyperhidrosis is a skin disorder that causes excessive sweating and is known to significantly impair quality of life.
- Primary hyperhidrosis is most often focal, affecting the palms, soles, and axillae; thighs, gluteal, and inguinal regions may also be involved. A patient may have one affected area or multiple focal sites of hyperhidrosis occurring simultaneously.
- Approximately 2.8% of the US population is affected by hyperhidrosis.
- Secondary hyperhidrosis is usually caused by an underlying medical condition or drug.
- Secondary hyperhidrosis must be ruled out before a diagnosis of primary hyperhidrosis is made.

INTRODUCTION

Hyperhidrosis is a skin disorder characterized by sweating in excess of what is required for thermoregulation. Hyperhidrosis can be primary or secondary in nature and may have general, regional, or focal manifestations.[1] Primary hyperhidrosis is most often focal and generally causes idiopathic, symmetrically bilateral excessive sweating of the axillae, palms, soles, or craniofacial region.[2,3] Secondary hyperhidrosis manifests most often as generalized excessive sweating that is related to an underlying medical condition or use of medication. Hyperhidrosis results in a decrease in quality of life, may cause impairment in the ability to carry out daily functions, and in some cases may increase risk of cutaneous infection.[4,5] Previous reports indicate that this condition affects 7.8 million people in the United States but this number may be conservative, because hyperhidrosis is both underreported by patients and underdiagnosed by health care professionals.[2]

Understanding the epidemiology of the disorder is critical for screening, diagnosis, and treatment.

PRIMARY HYPERHIDROSIS

Primary focal hyperhidrosis is excessive sweating in a specific region of the body that is not caused by other medical conditions or medications.[2] The cause of primary hyperhidrosis is not well understood, but is thought to be due to an overactivity of the autonomic nervous system. Eccrine sweat glands, which are located in the deep dermal layer of the skin, are innervated by post-ganglionic sympathetic nerve fibers and are stimulated by the neurotransmitter acetylcholine.[6] In primary hyperhidrosis, it is believed that these sweat glands receive aberrant stimulation by the sympathetic fibers causing excessive sweat production, although this has not been proved. Histologic evaluation of the affected areas demonstrates normal appearing eccrine sweat glands with a normal number, size, and density of the glands. Quantity

Financial Disclosures: There are no financial disclosures to report for any of the authors.
[a] Hennepin County Medical Center, 701 Park Avenue, Minneapolis, MN 55415, USA; [b] School of Medicine and Public Health, University of Wisconsin-Madison, 750 Highland Avenue, Madison, WI 53705, USA; [c] RidgeView Dermatology, 101 Candlewood Court, Lynchburg, VA 24502, USA
* Corresponding author.
E-mail addresses: hillsa1@gmail.com; sehill@ridgeviewdermatology.com

and function of acetylcholinesterase is also known to be normal, indicating an overabundance of neurotransmitter is not the cause.[3,6–8]

Focal Sites

Common focal sites for primary hyperhidrosis include palms, soles, axillae, craniofacial area, inguinal area, and gluteal region. Palmar, plantar, and axillary hyperhidrosis are the most comment manifestations of the disease.[2] Patients with primary hyperhidrosis may have one or multiple sites of involvement. For example, a patient may have palmar hyperhidrosis alone, palmar and axillary hyperhidrosis, or various other combinations of focal involvement.[2,9] This form of hyperhidrosis should be distinguished from generalized hyperhidrosis, and diagnostic criteria for focal hyperhidrosis can be helpful in accomplishing this. Whatever the manifestation of primary hyperhidrosis, the sweating is not related to another condition, but is itself the medical problem.[9]

Hexsel's Hyperhidrosis

Hexsel's hyperhidrosis is a type of regional primary hyperhidrosis that is characterized by chronic excessive sweating typically found in the inguinal region, including the medial surfaces of the upper thighs, suprapubic area, external genitalia, and at times the gluteal folds and gluteal cleft.[10] Patients with this condition have difficulty concealing the often-embarrassing sweat-drenched clothing in this area that typically results from having the disorder. Prevalence is largely unknown due to underreporting, but the condition appears less frequently than other forms of focal hyperhidrosis. Fifty percent of patients with Hexsel's hyperhidrosis have a positive family history of some form of hyperhidrosis, suggesting an inherited mechanism.[10]

Localized Unilateral Hyperhidrosis

Localized unilateral hyperhidrosis is usually seen as a sharply demarcated region of sweating on the forearm or forehead restricted to less than 10 cm by 10 cm. Most cases are idiopathic with no known triggering factors. The pathogenesis is unclear,[11] and one case report suggests that there is a hypohidrotic element to the disorder.[12] Less than 40 cases have been reported in the literature.[13]

Diagnostic Criteria for Primary Hyperhidrosis

Criteria for diagnosing primary focal hyperhidrosis include focal, visible, and excessive sweating for greater than 6 months without apparent cause with 2 or more of the following criteria: sweating that is bilateral and relatively symmetric, impairment of daily activities, frequency of at least one episode per week, age of onset less than 25 years, positive family history, and cessation of focal sweating during sleep.[14,15] A more recent analysis found that increasing the required criteria from 3 of 7 elements to 4 of 7 elements increases specificity (82% vs 21%) and positive predictive value (99% vs 95%). Increasing the specificity and positive predictive value further helps practitioners accurately delineate primary from secondary hyperhidrosis.[1] Primary hyperhidrosis that is truly generalized is rare, and the diagnosis should only be made after causes of secondary sweating are excluded. **Table 1** summarizes the criteria for diagnosis of hyperhidrosis.

Hyperhidrosis Prevalence

A major study seeking to determine the prevalence of hyperhidrosis in the United States was conducted wherein 150,000 US households were sent a survey inquiring about excessive sweating. Results from the survey projected that 2.8% of the US population is affected by hyperhidrosis.[2] Women and men were affected equally. Of those individuals affected, 50.8% have hyperhidrosis of the axillae, a third of whom described this condition as barely tolerable or intolerable and always or frequently interfering with daily activities.[2] The study also revealed that only 38% of respondents had ever discussed excessive sweating with a health care professional, with women being more likely than men to have discussed the problem (47.5% vs 28.6%). These findings demonstrate that although hyperhidrosis quite negatively affects quality of life, patients may be uncomfortable asking about this topic.[2] Hyperhidrosis is potentially underdiagnosed and undertreated; making this diagnosis necessitates inquiry during a routine review of systems regarding sweating and how it affects the patient's quality of life.

Although Strutton and colleagues[2] found a discrepancy between men and women in the reporting of sweating, no difference in incidence was found between the genders. Two studies of populations abroad, however, found that men had a higher incidence of hyperhidrosis: 16.66% versus 10.66% in Japan[16] and 18.1% versus 13.3% in Germany.[17] A study of Polish students found that men reported a higher intensity of hyperhidrosis symptoms than did women,[18] but a contradictory study in Canadian patients found that women reported being more severely affected.[19] Men are more likely to complain of craniofacial hyperhidrosis and to have "additional areas" involved (ie, back, chest, abdomen, forearm, genital, and lower

Table 1
Criteria for diagnosis

Primary Hyperhidrosis	1. Focal, visible, and excessive sweating of at least 6-mo duration without apparent cause 2. At least 2 of the following: • Bilateral and relatively symmetric • Impairs daily activities • At least one episode per week • Age of onset <25 y • Family history of hyperhidrosis • Cessation of focal sweating during sleep 3. Exclusion of secondary causes of excessive sweating
Secondary Generalized Hyperhidrosis	1. Generalized excessive sweating attributable to a definitive underlying medical cause; most commonly drugs, substance abuse, cardiovascular disorders, respiratory failure, infections, malignancies, endocrine/metabolic disorders, or neurologic disease.
Secondary Regional Hyperhidrosis	1. Localized anhidrosis with compensatory excessive sweating in other areas. 2. Identification of a definitive underlying cause; most commonly stroke, peripheral nerve damage, spinal cord lesion, neuropathy, or Ross syndrome.
Secondary Focal Hyperhidrosis	1. Excessive sweating in typical anatomic sites (palms, soles, axillae, craniofacial) or in a well-defined anatomic distribution (trunk, inguinal folds, buttocks, legs, submammary folds, neck, or wrist). 2. Identification of a definitive underlying cause; most commonly Frey syndrome, eccrine nevus, social anxiety disorder, neurologic disorder, or tumor.

Adapted from Walling HW. Clinical differentiation of primary from secondary hyperhidrosis. J Am Acad Dermatol 2011;64(4):693.

extremities).[19] Women are more likely to experience axillary hyperhidrosis.[4]

Hyperhidrosis Epidemiology

A retrospective chart review in 2011 found that 93% of patients with hyperhidrosis had primary disease, as opposed to secondary hyperhidrosis. More than 90% of patients with primary hyperhidrosis had a typical distribution, involving the axillae, palms, soles, and craniofacial areas.[1] Of these, the majority had an isolated axillary distribution (29%) or palms and soles distribution (25%); other patterns were isolated soles (15.5%), axillae with palms and soles (11%), palms (6%), and craniofacial (5%). Atypical distributions included the trunk (3%), inguinal folds (1.3%), buttocks, legs, submammary folds, neck, and wrist (<1% each).[1]

The onset of primary hyperhidrosis is most commonly between 14 and 25 years of age. Eccrine sweat glands are fully functional at birth, however, so hyperhidrosis is also seen in infants and young children. When the condition is seen in prepubertal individuals, it is generally the palmar or plantar variety that manifests (88.9%), with less likely presentations in the axillary (15.5%), facial (6.6%), or abdominal and dorsal (4.4%) regions.[20] A post-pubertal onset is more frequently associated with an axillary distribution.[19] The low prevalence of hyperhidrosis among the elderly is thought to possibly represent regression of the disease over time.

There is a positive family history in 35% to 56% of patients with hyperhidrosis; the pattern of inheritance is most likely autosomal dominant with variable penetrance.[2,4,19] Recently it has been reported that there may be a genetic linkage to chromosome 14.[9] Much like the overall prevalence of hyperhidrosis, the incidence of a positive family history is likely underestimated, because patients may conceal the presence of hyperhidrosis from family members due to embarrassment. In fact, one study found an even higher correlation with positive family history in patients with primary palmar hyperhidrosis, with 65% of patients having a positive family history.[21] Earlier age of onset (<20 years old) was also shown to correlate with positive family history, but these data may be confounded by the fact that patients with more severe cases present earlier.[19] **Box 1** summarizes these epidemiologic findings.

SECONDARY GENERALIZED HYPERHIDROSIS

Secondary generalized hyperhidrosis is excessive sweating that is caused by a medical condition or medication. Underlying conditions that may cause secondary hyperhidrosis can be physiologic, such as pregnancy, menopause, fever, excessive heat, or pathologic, including malignancy, carcinoid syndrome, hyperthyroidism, pheochromocytoma, tuberculosis, HIV, endocarditis, and autonomic dysreflexia, among others.[1,22,23] Drugs that are known to cause secondary hyperhidrosis include antidepressants, hypoglycemic agents, triptans, antipyretics, cholinergics, sympathomimetic agents, and many others. Secondary causes of hyperhidrosis must be ruled out before diagnosing primary hyperhidrosis.[2,14,22] This is most easily accomplished with a thorough review of systems and additional work-up as appropriate based on the patient response. Psychiatric disorders can also present with hyperhidrosis. Secondary hyperhidrosis is a clinical feature of 32% of people with social anxiety disorder.[24,25] Some debate exists, however, over whether the relationship between these 2 entities is causal.[26]

Clinical characteristics that help distinguish between primary and secondary types of hyperhidrosis include onset of the disease, characteristics of the sweating, and associated symptoms.[1] Patients with secondary hyperhidrosis are more likely to have onset older than 25 years compared with patients with primary hyperhidrosis. Although patients with primary hyperhidrosis are much more likely to have sweating in a typical distribution, those with secondary hyperhidrosis are significantly more likely to exhibit unilateral or asymmetrical sweating, to be generalized rather than focal, and to have symptoms during sleep ("night sweats"). Secondary hyperhidrosis is less often

associated with positive family history.[1] A middle-aged patient presenting with new onset generalized or asymmetrical sweating that also occurs while sleeping is highly suspicious for secondary hyperhidrosis. **Table 2** compares the characteristics of primary versus secondary hyperhidrosis.

SECONDARY FOCAL HYPERHIDROSIS

Although cases are considered rare, multiple types of focal secondary hyperhidrosis exist. For example, gustatory sweating is a condition wherein facial sweating occurs related to the consumption of foods. Gustatory sweating can be classified as either physiologic or nonphysiologic.[27,28] A physiologic type of gustatory sweating occurs as bilateral facial sweating that may occur in hot climates or after consumption of hot or spicy foods. Nonphysiologic types of gustatory sweating are caused by auriculotemporal nerve syndrome, diabetic neuropathy, infection, or sympathetic nerve damage from neoplasm or sympathectomy.[28] Frey syndrome is a focal facial sweating that occurs secondary to aberrant regeneration of damaged parasympathetic fibers that are destroyed by a parotid or salivary tumor or by surgical resection of a tumor. Frey syndrome may occur in up to 60% of patients after parotidectomy with facial nerve dissection.[28,29] Auriculotemporal nerve syndrome can also occur sporadically as a familial trait and in these cases, occurs without a preceding trauma to the nerve. Diabetic gustatory sweating may occur as a byproduct of sympathetic denervation, which is compensated for by innervation of aberrant parasympathetic fibers. These fibers stem from the minor petrous nerve and innervate the parotid gland, causing sweating when salivation is induced. This finding is seen in 69% of patients with diabetic nephropathy and 36% of patients with diabetic

Table 2
Characteristics of primary versus secondary hyperhidrosis

Comparison of Primary and Secondary Hyperhidrosis	
Primary Hyperhidrosis	**Secondary Hyperhidrosis**
• Sweating in a typical distribution • Positive family history	• Onset older than 25 y • Unilateral and/or symmetric • Generalized rather than focal • Presents nocturnally or during sleep

Table 3
Causes of secondary hyperhidrosis

Common Conditions	Nonneural Conditions
Acute febrile illness (eg, infection)	Arteriovenous fistula
Alcoholism	Blue rubber bleb nevus syndrome
Diabetes mellitus	Cold erythema
Gout	Drugs
Heart failure	Glomus tumors
Hyperthyroidism	Klippel-Trenaunay syndrome
Lymphoma	Local heat
Menopause	Maffucci syndrome
Obesity	Organoid and sudoriparous nevi
Parkinson disease	
Pregnancy	
Rheumatoid arthritis	

Nervous System–Mediated Conditions: A,B,C, D

Hypothalamic conditions (mediated by the hypothalamus)(A)
 Carcinoid syndrome
 Cardiac shock
 Chédiak-Higashi syndrome
 Chronic arsenic intoxication
 Cold injury
 Debility
 Chronic infection (eg, tuberculosis, malaria, brucellosis)
 Drugs
 Familial dysautonomia
 Erythrocyanosis
 Essential hyperhidrosis
 Exercise
 Hines-Bannick syndrome
 Hyperpituitarism
 Hypoglycemia
 Hypothalamic mass
 Idiopathic unilateral circumscribed hyperhidrosis
 Infantile scurvy
 Pheochromocytoma
 POEMS syndrome
 Porphyria
 Post-encephalitis
 Raynaud phenomenon or disease
 Reflex sympathetic dystrophy
 Rickets
 Stroke/cerebrovascular accident/transient ischemic attack (affecting hypothalamus)
 Symmetric lividity of the palms and soles
 Vitiligo
Peripheral-reflexive conditions (B)
 Drugs/medications
 Perilesional (eg, burn)
Cortical conditions (mediated by the cerebral cortex) (C)
 Congenital autonomic dysfunction with universal pain loss
 Congenital ichthyosiform erythroderma
 Epidermolysis bullosa simplex
 Familial dysautonomia
 Gorlin syndrome
 Palmoplantar keratoderma
 Pachyonychia congenita
 Pressure and postural hyperhidrosis
Medullary/Spinal conditions (mediated by the medulla oblongata or spinal nerves) (D)
 Auriculotemporal syndrome
 Granulosis rubra nasi
 Physiologic gustatory sweating
 Post-traumatic (spinal cord transection or thoracic sympathetic chain injury)
 Encephalitis
 Sytingomyelia

Box 2
Drugs that cause hyperhidrosis

Pain Medications

- Celebrex
- Hydrocodone/Vicodin
- Toradol/Ketoralac
- Morphine
- Relafen/Nabumetone
- Naproxen/Aleve
- Oxycodone/Roxicodone
- Ultram/Tramadol
- Duragesic/Fentanyl
- Marinol

Heart/Blood Pressure

- Norvasc/Amlodipine
- Lotensin/Benazepril
- Bumex/Bumetanide
- Coreg/Carvedilol
- Digoxin/Lanoxin
- Persantine/Dipyridamole
- Cardura/Doxazosin
- Vasotec/Enalapril
- Hydralazine
- Prinivil/Zestril/Lisinopril
- Cozaar/Losartan
- Lopressor/Metoprolol
- Nifedipine/Procardia
- Rythmol/Propafenone
- Altace/Ramipril
- Calan/Verapamil

Oncology/Cancer

- Arimidex/Anastrozole
- Lupron/Leuprolide
- Tamoxifen/Nolvadex

Gastrointestinal

- Lomotil/Diphenoxylate
- Anzemet/Dolasetron
- Asacol/Mesalamine
- Prilosec/Omeprazole
- Aciphex/Rabeprazole

Head/Neck Medications

- Aerobid/Nasarel
- Claritin/Loratadine
- Sudafed/Pseudoephedrine
- Aristocort/Azmacort
- Afrin/Neo-Synephrine
- Zinc tablets/Cold-EEZE

Hormonal/Endocrine

- Calcitonin/Fortical
- Glucotrol/Glipizide
- Insulin/Humulin
- Synthroid/Thyroid
- Depo-Provera
- Prednisolone/Orapred
- Evista/Raloxifene
- Genotropin/Somatropin
- Testosterone/Androgel
- Antibodies/Tositumomab
- Vasopressin/Pitressin

Skin Medications

- Topical steroids
- Accutane/Isotretinoin
- Lidocaine/Carbocaine
- Selsun/Selenium sulfide

Blood/Immune System

- Neoral/Cyclosporine
- Ferrous gluconate/Iron
- Remicade/Infliximab
- Cellcept/Mycophenolate
- Prograf/Tacrolimus

Antibiotics/Antivirals

- Acyclovir/Zovirax
- Rocephin/Ceftriaxone
- Cipro/Ciprofloxacin
- Sustiva/Efavirenz
- Foscavir/Foscarnet
- Tequin/Gatifloxacin
- Avelox/Moxifloxacin
- Ketek/Telithromycin
- Ribavirin/Copegus
- Retrovir/AZT

Psychiatric/Neuro Medications

- Elavil/Amitriptyline
- Buspar/Buspirone
- Tegretol/Carbamazepine
- Celexa/Citalopram
- Clozaril/Clozapine
- Norpramin/Desipramine
- Adderall/Amphetamine
- Migranal/Ergotamine
- Aricept/Donepezil
- Cymbalta/Duloxetine
- Lexapro/Escitalopram
- Lunesta/Eszopiclone
- Prozac/Fluoxetine
- Haldol/Haloperidol
- Sinemet/Levodopa
- Provigil/Modafinil

Eye Medications

- Phospholine Iodide
- Vascon/Naphazoline
- Alcaine/Vardenafil

Lung Medications

- Advair/Fluticasone
- Combivent/Ipratropium
- Xopenex/Levalbuterol
- Alupent/Metaproterenol

Genital/Urinary

- Cialis/Tadalafil
- Levitra/Vardenafil

Adapted from International Hyperhidrosis Society, Quakertown, PA; with permission.

neuropathy.[27] Gustatory sweating may also occur after infection, most commonly secondary to herpes zoster infection.[23]

Secondary focal hyperhidrosis may be seen in conjunction with a variety of cutaneous disorders, although a causal relationship is not established. Although uncommon, with only 20 reports in the literature, an eccrine nevus can cause localized hyperhidrosis in an area of skin with increased numbers of eccrine glands.[30] Associated hypertrichosis and comedones can be seen in the area. Another term used in the literature to describe an eccrine nevus is nevus sudoriferous.[31,32] A similar lesion, the eccrine angiomatous hamartoma,[33] shows an abundance of eccrine glands but is also accompanied by a proliferation of vascular channels. Fewer than 50 cases have been reported. Because of similarities in histologic appearance and make-up, these lesions may share a similar genetic pathway. Pachyonychia congenita is a rare autosomal dominant genodermatosis that is often associated with focal palmar and plantar hyperhidrosis. There have only been 450 reported cases of this since 1901. One study found hyperhidrosis in 51.5% of all patients with pachyonychia congenita and in 22.7% of children with the disorder.[34] Other associated disorders include palmoplantar keratodermas, glomus tumor, blue rubber bleb nevus syndrome, nevus sudoriferous, POEMS (polyneuropathy, organomegaly, endocrinopathy, M protein, skin changes) syndrome, speckled lentiginous nevus syndrome, Riley-Day syndrome, pachydermoperiostosis, Gopalan syndrome, causalgia, pretibial myxedema, Buerger disease, eccrine pilar angiomatous hamartoma, local injury, and increased size of eccrine glands.[13] **Table 3** summarizes the causes of secondary hyperhidrosis. **Box 2** lists drugs that can cause hyperhidrosis.

SECONDARY REGIONAL HYPERHIDROSIS

Secondary regional hyperhidrosis is often characterized by anhidrosis in one area with compensatory hyperhidrosis in another area. Most commonly the condition is iatrogenic, in the form of compensatory sweating following surgical treatment of primary focal hyperhidrosis. It may also manifest as part of Ross syndrome or in one of several neurologic conditions.[7,35,36]

Compensatory hyperhidrosis, sweating in areas remote from the original problem location, is a known potential complication of endoscopic thoracic sympathectomy (ETS). In 2011, expert consensus by the Society of Thoracic Surgeons reported that 3% to 98% of patients having had ETS develop iatrogenic compensatory hyperhidrosis.[37]

One large-scale study found only 55% of patients developed compensatory sweating, with 2% considering the compensatory hyperhidrosis to be as bothersome as the original symptoms.[38]

Ross syndrome is a rare nervous system disorder characterized by a tonic pupil ("Adie pupil"), deep tendon hyporeflexia, and unilateral or bilateral anhidrosis.[36] It can present with associated segmental hyperhidrosis. Recent studies suggest that Ross syndrome may be autoimmune in etiology.[35] The disorder is rare, with about 50 case reports in the literature.[39]

Secondary regional hyperhidrosis may be related to stroke, spinal cord lesion, neoplasm, or peripheral neuropathies.[40,41] One pathophysiologic explanation for this phenomenon is that the primary lesion causes impairment of preganglionic neurons and subsequent anhidrosis, but bladder distension and other visceral stimuli enter the spinal cord distal to the lesion, causing a spinal dysreflexia that manifests as abnormal sweating. The phenomenon has also been called "perilesionary hyperhidrosis" or "border-zone sweating".[40] One study evaluated 633 strokes and found hemihyperhidrosis in 6 patients, whereas another evaluated 350 strokes and found hemihyperhidrosis in 5 patients, so incidence of hyperhidrosis in cerebral infarction may be estimated at 1% to 2%.[42] Hyperhidrosis can also be associated with syringomyelia and other central nervous system diseases.[43]

SUMMARY

Understanding the epidemiology of hyperhidrosis can improve the diagnosis, treatment, and ideally the prognosis of the disorder. Because of the social implications of excessive sweating, hyperhidrosis is likely underreported and therefore undertreated. Providers who are knowledgeable about hyperhidrosis may be more likely to identify those who are suffering from the disorder and may be more comfortable beginning the delicate dialogue about how excessive sweating might be affecting the patient.

Although most patients suffer from primary hyperhidrosis, an accurate assessment must be made to rule out secondary causes of hyperhidrosis to tailor treatment appropriately. With a modest improvement in the recognition of hyperhidrosis, a provider has the opportunity to make a major impact on a patient's quality of life.

REFERENCES

1. Walling HW. Clinical differentiation of primary from secondary hyperhidrosis. J Am Acad Dermatol 2011;64(4):690–5.

2. Strutton DR, Kowalski JW, Glaser DA, et al. US prevalence of hyperhidrosis and impact on individuals with axillary hyperhidrosis: results from a national survey. J Am Acad Dermatol 2004;51:241–8.

3. Lowe N, Campanati A, Bodokh I, et al. The place of botulinum toxin type A in the treatment of focal hyperhidrosis. Br J Dermatol 2004;151:1115–22.

4. Walling HW. Primary hyperhidrosis increases the risk of cutaneous infection: a case control study of 387 patients. J Am Acad Dermatol 2009;61(2):242–6.

5. Naumann M, Hofmann U, Bergmann I, et al. Focal hyperhidrosis: effective treatment with intracutaneous botulinum toxin. Arch Dermatol 1998;134:301–4.

6. Solish N, Bertucci V, Dansereau A, et al. A comprehensive approach to the recognition, diagnosis and severity-based treatment of focal hyperhidrosis: recommendations of the Canadian hyperhidrosis advisory committee. Dermatol Surg 2007;33(8): 908–23.

7. Sato K, Ohtsuyama M, Samman G. Eccrine sweat gland disorders. J Am Acad Dermatol 1991;24(6): 1010–4.

8. Haider A, Solish N. Focal hyperhidrosis: diagnosis and management. CMAJ 2005;172(1):69–75.

9. Smith FC. Hyperhidrosis. Vasc Surg 2013;31(5): 251–5.

10. Hexsel DM, Dal'Forno T, Hexsel CL. Inguinal, or Hexsel's Hyperhidrosis. Clin Dermatol 2004;22:53–9.

11. Kreyden OP, Schmid-Grendelmeier P, Burg G. Idiopathic localized unilateral hyperhidrosis. Case report of successful treatment with Botulinum Toxin Type A and review of the literature. Arch Dermatol 2001;137:1622–5.

12. Kocyigit P, Akay BN, Saral S, et al. Unilateral hyperhidrosis with accompanying contralateral anhidrosis. Clin Exp Dermatol 2009;34:e544–6.

13. Baskan EM, Karli N, Baykara M, et al. Localized unilateral hyperhidrosis and neurofibromatosis type I: case report of a New Association. Dermatology 2005;211:286–9.

14. Hornberger J, Grimes K, Naumann M, et al. Recognition diagnosis, and treatment of primary focal hyperhidrosis. J Am Acad Dermatol 2004;51(2): 274–86.

15. Glaser DA, Herbert AA, Pariser DM, et al. Facial Hyperhidrosis: best practice recommendations and special considerations. Cutis 2007;79(5):29–32.

16. Fujimoto T, Kawahara K, Yokozeki H. Epidemiological study and considerations of primary focal hyperhidrosis in Japan: from questionnaire analysis. J Dermatol 2013;40:886–90.

17. Augustin M, Radtke MA, Herberger K, et al. Prevalence and disease burden of hyperhidrosis in the adult population. Dermatology 2013;227:10–3.

18. Stefaniak T, Tomaszewski KA, Proczko-Markuszewska M, et al. Is subjective hyperhidrosis assessment sufficient enough? Prevalence of hyperhidrosis among young Polish adults. J Dermatol 2013; 40:819–23.

19. Lear W, Kessler E, Solish N, et al. An epidemiological study of hyperhidrosis. Dermatol Surg 2007;33: S69–75.

20. Wolosker N, Schvartsman C, Krutman M, et al. Efficacy and quality of life outcomes of oxybutynin for treating palmar hyperhidrosis in children younger than 14 years old. Pediatr Dermatol 2014;31:48–53.

21. Ro KM, Cantor RM, Lange KL, et al. Palmar hyperhidrosis: evidence of genetic transmission. J Vasc Surg 2002;35(2):382–6.

22. Glaser DA, Herbert AA, Pariser DM, et al. Primary focal hyperhidrosis: scope of the problem. Cutis 2007;79(5):5–17.

23. Chopra KF, Evans T, Severson J, et al. Acute varicella zoster with postherpetic hyperhidrosis as the initial presentation of HIV infection. J Am Acad Dermatol 1999;41:119–21.

24. Connor KM, Cook JL, Davidson JR. Botulinum toxin treatment of social anxiety disorder with hyperhidrosis: a placebo-controlled double-blind trial. J Clin Psychiatry 2006;67:30–6.

25. Davidson JR, Foa EB, Connor KM, et al. Hyperhidrosis in social anxiety disorder. Prog Neuropsychopharmacol Biol Psychiatry 2002;26:1327–31.

26. Ruchinskas R. Hyperhidrosis and anxiety: chicken or egg? Dermatology 2007;214:195–6.

27. Shaw JE, Parker R, Hollis S, et al. Gustatory sweating in diabetes mellitus. Diabet Med 1996;13: 1033–7.

28. Blair D, Sagel J, Taylor I. Diabetic gustatory sweating. South Med J 2002;95(3):360–2.

29. de Bree R, van der Waal I, Leemans R. Management of Frey syndrome. Head Neck 2007;29(8):773–8. Wiley InterScience: epublished.

30. Dua J, Grabczynska S. Eccrine nevus affecting the forearm of an 11-year-old girl successfully controlled with topical glycopyrrolate. Pediatr Dermatol 2013;1–2.

31. Kawaoka JC, Gray J, Schappell D, et al. Eccrine nevus. J Am Acad Dermatol 2004;51:301–4.

32. Goldstein N. Ephidrosis (local hyperhidrosis). Nevus sudoriferous. Arch Dermatol 1967;96(1):67–8.

33. Sen S, Chatterjee G, Mitra PK, et al. Eccrine angiomatous naevus revisited. Indian J Dermatol 2012; 57(4):313–5.

34. Shah S, Boen M, Kenner-Bell B, et al. Pachyonychia congenital in pediatric patients: natural history, features and impact. JAMA Dermatol 2014;150(2): 146–53. epublished: E1–7.

35. Biju V, Sawhney MP, Vishal S. Ross syndrome with ANA positivity: a clue to possible autoimmune origin and treatment with intravenous immunoglobulin. Indian J Dermatol 2010;55(3):274–6.

36. Ballestero-Diez M, Garcia-Rio I, Dauden E, et al. Ross Syndrome, and entity included within the spectrum of partial disautonomic syndromes. J Eur Acad Dermatol Venereol 2005;19:729–31.

37. Cerfolio RJ, Milanez de Campos JR, Bryant AS, et al. The society of thoracic surgeons expert consensus for the surgical treatment of hyperhidrosis. Ann Thorac Surg 2011;91:1642–8.

38. Drott C, Gothberg G, Claes G. Endoscopic transthoracic sympathectomy: an efficient and safe method for the treatment of hyperhidrosis. J Am Acad Dermatol 1995;33:78–81.

39. Yazar S, Aslan C, Serdar ZA, et al. Ross syndrome: Unilateral hyperhidrosis, Adie's tonic pupils and diffuse areflexia. J Dtsch Dermatol Ges 2010;8:1004–6.

40. Saito H, Sakuma H, Seno K. A case of traumatic high thoracic myelopathy presenting dissociated impairment of rostral sympathetic innervations and isolated segmental sweating on otherwise anhidrotic trunk. J Exp Med 1999;188:95–102.

41. Nishimura J, Tamada Y, Iwase S, et al. A case of lung cancer with unilateral anhidrosis and contralateral hyperhidrosis as the first clinical manifestation. J Am Acad Dermatol 2011;65(2):438–40.

42. Faruqi S, Redmond G, Ram P, et al. Hemihyperhidrosis in cerebral infarction. Age Ageing 2004;33: 514–5.

43. Smith CD. A hypothalamic stroke producing recurrent hemihyperhidrosis. Neurology 2001;56: 1394–6.

Impact of Hyperhidrosis on Quality of Life and its Assessment

Henning Hamm, MD

KEYWORDS

- Hyperhidrosis • Impact • Quality of life • Dermatology Life Quality Index
- Hyperhidrosis Disease Severity Scale • Hyperhidrosis Impact Questionnaire • Botulinum toxin
- Endoscopic thoracic sympathectomy

KEY POINTS

- Primary focal hyperhidrosis severely affects many aspects of daily life including emotional well-being, interpersonal relationships, leisure activities, personal hygiene, work and productivity, and self-esteem.
- For evaluation of its impact on patients, disease-specific questionnaires, such as the Hyperhidrosis Disease Severity Scale, the Clinical Protocol for Quality of Life, and the comprehensive Hyperhidrosis Impact Questionnaire, have been developed.
- Limitations of hyperhidrosis as a dermatologic condition are commonly measured by the Dermatology Life Quality Index. The 36-item Short Form Health Survey is the most established instrument for recording the impairment of general health-related quality of life in patients with hyperhidrosis.
- Assessment of quality of life in patients with primary focal hyperhidrosis has particularly been used to prove the substantial benefits of endoscopic thoracic sympathectomy and botulinum toxin treatment.

INTRODUCTION

It has been known for a long time that hyperhidrosis is a stigmatizing condition that may severely affect many aspects of daily life including emotional well-being, interpersonal relationships, leisure activities, personal hygiene, work and productivity, and self-esteem. In 1977, Adar and colleagues[1] pointed out that hyperhidrosis caused considerable social, professional, and emotional embarrassment in their patients with primary palmar hyperhidrosis (PPH), and claimed that sympathectomy led to improved quality of life (QoL). The first time the term QoL in context with

hyperhidrosis appeared in the heading of a medical publication was in a short comment on therapeutic options in the Swedish medical journal *Läkartidningen*.[2] However, serious efforts to scientifically evaluate the impact of hyperhidrosis on patients lasted until the turn of the century after endoscopic thoracic sympathectomy (ETS) and injections of botulinum toxin were introduced in the therapeutic armamentarium of primary focal hyperhidrosis (PFH).

General limitations caused by PFH include feelings of embarrassment, shame, insecurity, frustration, unhappiness, and depression. Patients often have a low self-esteem and lack of

Disclosure Statement: The author has been investigator in clinical trials sponsored by Allergan Co, United Kingdom, and Ipsen Pharma GmbH, Germany. He has received grants from Allergan Co for hyperhidrosis research and has been a consultant for Pharm-Allergan GmbH, Germany. He has received speaker's honoraria from Allergan and from the International Hyperhidrosis Society.
Department of Dermatology, Venereology and Allergology, University Hospital Würzburg, Josef-Schneider-Straße 2, D-97080 Würzburg, Germany
E-mail address: hamm_h@ukw.de

Dermatol Clin 32 (2014) 467–476
http://dx.doi.org/10.1016/j.det.2014.06.004
0733-8635/14/$ – see front matter © 2014 Elsevier Inc. All rights reserved.

self-confidence. Difficulties with social and intimate relationships may lead to reclusiveness and avoidance of social interactions and leisure activities. Individual patients may even perceive suicidal ideation. Moreover, patients may experience functional restraints and may be compelled to adapt their behavior depending on whether axillae, palms, soles, or other sites are involved. For example, patients with primary axillary hyperhidrosis (PAH) spend much time and energy on their personal hygiene, whereas PPH often results in occupational impairment.[3] Further site-related handicaps are summarized in **Box 1**. In addition, PFH markedly increases site-specific risks of cutaneous infection, especially pitted keratolysis, dermatophytosis, and vulgar/plantar warts.[4] The detriments of affected patients may be exacerbated by low awareness of PFH as a treatable medical condition and the little importance given to the patient's complaints by others.

This article gives an overview on attempts to substantiate the various limitations induced by PFH beyond objectively verifiable measurement of sweat production and delineation of the hyperhidrotic area by the Minor iodine starch test. Questionnaires used for evaluation are classified into disease-specific instruments, those devoted to common limitations in dermatologic conditions, and those measuring general health-related QoL or certain aspects of impairment. With few exceptions, QoL assessment in hyperhidrosis has been used to prove the efficacy of therapeutic interventions, such as ETS, botulinum toxin treatment, and more recently oral anticholinergic drugs.

DISEASE-SPECIFIC ASSESSMENT OF QoL
Hyperhidrosis Disease Severity Scale

The Hyperhidrosis Disease Severity Scale (HDSS) is a single-item question allowing 4 gradations of the tolerability of sweating and its interference with daily activities (**Table 1**). This simple, validated diagnostic tool offers a quick way to estimate the impairment of QoL caused by sweating. A score of 3 or 4 indicates severe hyperhidrosis, a score of 2 moderate hyperhidrosis, and a score of 1 absence of hyperhidrosis.

The HDSS was introduced in 2004 to determine the prevalence of hyperhidrosis in the United States from a representative sample of 150,000 households.[5] The overall prevalence of hyperhidrosis was estimated at 2.8% in the general population, the prevalence of axillary hyperhidrosis at 1.4%, and the prevalence of severe axillary hyperhidrosis corresponding with HDSS scores 3 or 4 at 0.5%.

In a large prospective open-label study in 142 Canadian patients with PAH treated with botulinum neurotoxin type A (BoNT/A), HDSS scores

---

Box 1
Selection of site-specific handicaps caused by PFH

Primary axillary and inguinal hyperhidrosis

- Soaking, staining, and soiling of clothing
- Restriction in the choice of clothing
- Need for frequent showering and change of clothing

Primary palmar hyperhidrosis

- Difficulties in manual activities and in handling objects, such as in writing, drawing, playing musical instruments, knitting, car driving, opening doorknobs, and handling balls in sports
- Dropping of glass objects from hands
- Soiling of paper and artwork
- Avoidance of hand shaking
- Electrical shocks to moist hands in mechanics and electricians
- Corrosion of metal objects
- Need for wiping hands dry

Primary plantar hyperhidrosis

- Soaking, staining, and destruction of shoes
- Difficulties in wearing sandals, slippers, and flip-flops
- Difficulties when walking barefoot
- Need for wearing absorbing socks

Primary craniofacial hyperhidrosis

- Dripping of sweat drops on objects or persons when bent forward
- Soaking of collars
- Need for wiping scalp and face dry

Table 1
The Hyperhidrosis Disease Severity Scale

Question: How Would You Rate the Severity of Your Hyperhidrosis?	Score
My sweating is never noticeable and never interferes with my daily activities	1
My sweating is tolerable but sometimes interferes with my daily activities	2
My sweating is barely tolerable and frequently interferes with my daily activities	3
My sweating is intolerable and always interferes with my daily activities	4

of 3 or 4 served as inclusion criteria.[6] Four weeks after treatment, 85% of patients were classified as treatment responders achieving an HDSS score of 1 or 2, and 59% of patients noted complete resolution of their symptoms, as indicated by an HDSS score of 1. Only patients with PAH with HDSS scores of 3 and 4 were included in a US placebo-controlled study on the efficacy and safety of 2 different doses of BoNT/A (75 U or 50 U per axilla).[7] An improvement of at least 2 points in HDSS score from baseline 4 weeks after the first treatment was indicated by 75% of subjects in both the BoNT/A 75-U and 50-U groups compared with 25% of subjects in the placebo group.

Site-specific HDSS scores were obtained in 152 patients with severe PPH before and about 1 year after ETS in order to compare clamping versus cutting of the sympathetic nerve at the T3 level.[8] No significant differences were found. Campanati and colleagues[9] examined the relapse-free survival in 41 patients with PPH and 38 patients with PAH treated with BoNT/A. Relapse was defined as 2-point worsening of the achieved HDSS score. Duration of the therapeutic effect was not significantly influenced by disease-related QoL impairment before treatment. In a German randomized, placebo-controlled study on the efficacy and safety of methantheline bromide in 339 patients affected by PAH and palmar-axillary hyperhidrosis, the mean HDSS scores decreased after 4 weeks in the verum group from 3.2 to 2.4 compared with 3.2 to 2.7 for placebo.[10] The HDSS was used to intraindividually compare the effectiveness of suction curettage to 1 axilla and BoNT/A injections to the contralateral side in 20 patients with PAH.[11] Toxin injections induced a larger decrease in HDSS scores than surgery at 3 and 6 months after intervention.

In recommendations for the treatment of PFH the Canadian Hyperhidrosis Advisory Committee pointed out the HDSS as a valuable method to tailor treatment based on disease severity.[12] The investigators defined treatment success as an improvement from an HDSS score of 4 or 3 to a score of 2 or 1 or from a score of 2 to 1. Treatment failure was defined as no change in HDSS score after 1 month of therapy or lack of tolerability for the treatment.

The HDSS also showed the effectiveness of BoNT/A treatment in severe compensatory hyperhidrosis of the trunk[13] and of oral oxybutynin in postmenopausal hyperhidrosis.[14]

Similar to the HDSS, the Quality of Life Index is a single-item question rating the impact of the disease on QoL on a scale from 0 (no effect) to 3 (major/significant effect).[15,16]

Amir–de Campos Clinical Protocol for QoL

In 2000, Amir and colleagues[17] described the development of a short, disease-specific questionnaire for assessment of the impact of PFH relying on in-depth interviews with patients. Based on this preliminary tool, de Campos and colleagues[18] devised an instrument, later termed the Clinical Protocol for Quality of Life, and applied it to 378 patients with predominantly PPH before and at least 30 days after ETS. The investigators noted a much better QoL in 75.7% and a slightly better QoL in 10.7% of patients after surgery.

The questionnaire includes 1 general question asking for overall QoL reduction and 20 questions belonging to 4 domains covering compromising effects on (manual) function and social activities (writing, manual work, leisure, sports, hand shaking, socializing in public places, grasping objects, social dancing), personal limitations with the partner (holding hands, intimate touching, intimate affairs), emotional impairment (need for justification, feeling of rejection by others) and restrictions under special circumstances (in closed or hot environment, when tense or worried, when thinking about the problem, before an examination/meeting/speaking in front of people, when wearing sandals/walking barefoot, when wearing colored clothes, when having problems at school/work). Every question has 5 levels of response displayed in a table with only 1 answer allowed. The summed total score may range from 20 to 100, with higher levels indicating greater severity and poorer QoL. The result may be ranked to one of 5 levels of QoL impairment (total score 84–100, very poor QoL; 68 to 83, poor QoL; 52–67, good QoL; 36–51, very good QoL; and 20–35, excellent QoL). Improvement of QoL after treatment is rated accordingly.

Since this original publication, the protocol has been extensively used by the São Paulo group of vascular and thoracic surgeons[19–27] and some other investigators[28–32] to prove the efficacy of ETS in PFH. In a large retrospective analysis of 453 patients with PPH and PAH, Wolosker and colleagues[26] found that the QoL had improved in 90.9% of patients around 30 days after surgery and that this effect was sustained in almost all of them until the fifth postoperative year. Stable amelioration of QoL as measured by the Amir–de Campos and the Keller protocols (discussed later) 5 years after ETS surgery for upper limb hyperhidrosis was confirmed in 174 Austrian patients provided that compensatory sweating and recurrence were not severe.[32] Another evaluation by the São Paulo group revealed that 855 patients with very poor QoL scores before ETS surgery benefited on average much more in terms of QoL improvement than 312 patients with poor QoL.[24] The same result was observed for both the PPH and PAH subgroups. There were no significant differences between genders with regard to QoL improvement.[23] Differences that were similarly small were evident when comparing the outcome after different methods of surgery[30] or intervention at distinct ganglion denervation levels.[19,21,22,25] The variable postoperative degree of compensatory hyperhidrosis depending on the level of surgery was not always reflected in the results of QoL assessment by this protocol.[19]

One study comparing the effects of ETS and BoNT/A injections in PPH showed quick and similarly strong improvement of QoL scores in both groups.[29] After 6 months, QoL had mildly worsened in the surgical group and there was a more marked decreased in patients treated with BoNT/A.

In recent years, Wolosker and colleagues[33–37] extended the use of the Amir–de Campos protocol to the evaluation of the initial treatment of patients with PPH and PAH with the oral anticholinergic drug oxybutynin. After 12 weeks, QoL improvement was noted in approximately 70% of patients, with dry mouth being virtually the only adverse effect. An adapted version of the protocol with total scores ranging from 17 to 85 was applied to 45 children with PPH aged 7 to 14 years.[38] The median QoL total score decreased from 73 before to 36 after 6 weeks of oxybutynin treatment, and reduction was noted in 70% of patients. Best responses were seen in children with very poor pretreatment QoL.

Hyperhidrosis Impact Questionnaire

Hyperhidrosis characteristics, use of medical resources, and functional limitations in daily activities caused by hyperhidrosis are explored by the Hyperhidrosis Impact Questionnaire (HHIQ).[3] The 41-item instrument was developed by collaborators of the University Hospital Würzburg and Allergan and is based on a thorough literature review and on qualitative interviews with physicians and ex-patients of our outpatient hyperhidrosis clinic.[39] The validated questionnaire includes items on disease characteristics, use of medical resources, employment and productivity, various daily activities, and psychological and emotional well-being. Each item is individually scored.

In a large study on 345 patients with PFH, mainly PAH and PPH, compared with 154 healthy controls, 63% of affected patients reported that they were moderately to extremely limited at work, and 44% reported that their sweating resulted in moderate to extreme impairment of their effectiveness at work.[3] Almost half of the patients (42%) claimed that their sweating had prevented them from following a particular career path. Nearly three-quarters of patients with hyperhidrosis (74%) complained of being emotionally damaged or injured to a moderate to extreme degree. Most patients reported feeling less confident than they would like (74%) and to be unhappy or depressed (63%), with a higher proportion of axillary than palmar patients (71% vs 54%). Many patients reported being moderately to extremely limited in social situations such as meeting people for the first time (71%), in developing personal relationships (59%), in participating in family events or spending time with friends (54%), and in sexual activities (34%). As expected, patients with PPH were significantly more limited in shaking hands than those with PAH (97% vs 33%), whereas patients with PAH were more limited in staying in public places (65% vs 45%). Significantly more patients with PAH than with PPH reported decreasing their leisure time (59% vs 41%) and missing activities with family and friends (59% vs 41%). With regard to physical impairment, more patients with PAH than with PPH changed their clothes at least twice a day (70% vs 31%), spent at least 15 minutes per day treating their symptoms (38% vs 22%), and showered or bathed at least twice daily (27% vs 10%).

Parts of the HHIQ were used in the investigation of the US prevalence of hyperhidrosis.[5] People with axillary hyperhidrosis and HDSS scores of 3 and 4 most frequently indicated moderate to extreme limitations in meeting people (46.7%), in romantic/intimate situations (46.0%), in sports (45.9%), being in public places (45.8%), and in developing personal relationships (37.0%). Most of them reported reduced self-confidence (69.8%), frustration with certain daily activities (58.2%), and feeling unhappy (54.8%).

The questionnaire was also applied to the participants of several large placebo-controlled studies on the effectiveness of BoNT/A treatment in PAH.[6,40,41] In contrast with placebo groups, limitations in personal relationships and social situations, reduction of the performance and productivity at work, and impact of the disease on the emotional status improved significantly after BoNT/A injections. The most dramatic changes were noted in the ability to perform daily tasks and work activities and in the degree of limitation on being in public places, on meeting people for the first time, and on developing personal relationships.[6,40,41]

Other Hyperhidrosis-specific Instruments

Keller and colleagues[42] introduced a scale with a series of 15 questions addressing the common physical symptoms and social stigmata associated with PFH in daily life. Five questions address problems of palmar sweating in certain situations, such as shaking hands, writing an examination, initiating intimate contact, driving a car, and wearing gloves. Likewise, 5 questions each reflect limitations caused by excessive axillary and plantar sweating. The Keller scale has repeatedly been used by thoracic surgeons from Vienna to prove the beneficial effect of ETS.[32,43–45] In addition, this group tried to quantify the severity of sweating before and after surgery by a visual analog scale graded between 0 (no symptoms) and 10 (worst possible symptom) (the Hyperhidrosis Index). Postoperative results were better in patients with PPH than in those with PAH and much better than in patients with primary plantar hyperhidrosis.[43,44] QoL improvement, as assessed by the Keller scale, was also shown in 36 patients with PFH treated with oral glycopyrrolate.[31]

A large number of investigators preferred self-made disease-specific questionnaires for QoL evaluation before and after treatment, in most instances ETS.[8,46–65] Interviews by telephone or e-mail were sometimes done to complete missing answers. Detailed information for the issues covered by the particular questionnaires is beyond the scope of this article and is presented in only some of the articles.[49–52,58,61] Only rarely, attempts to verify the validity and reliability of the instruments are described,[47] putting their general usefulness into question.

DERMATOLOGY-RELATED ASSESSMENT OF QoL
Dermatology Life Quality Index

The Dermatology Life Quality Index (DLQI) developed by Finlay and Khan[66] in 1994 is the most frequently used instrument to measure the effects of dermatologic diseases on QoL. The simple, validated questionnaire consists of 10 items covering 6 domains: symptoms and feelings, daily activities, leisure, work and school, personal relationships, and treatment. Each item has 4 gradations (3, very much; 2, a lot; 1, a little; 0, not at all/not relevant). Total scores range from 0 to 30, with higher scores indicating greater impairment.

In our study, the 345 patients with PFH had a mean DLQI total score of 9.2.[3] Patients with PAH had a score of 10.0 and those with PPH had a score of 8.8, compared with 0.7 in healthy controls. Greatest impairments were observed for the daily activities and symptoms/feelings domains. The mean daily activities score was significantly higher in patients with PAH than in

patients with PPH, whereas the latter had significantly higher mean treatment scores.

Investigators from Sweden were the first to use the DLQI for assessing QoL before and after treatment.[67] In 58 patients treated with BoNT/A for PPH, PAH, and plantar hyperhidrosis they noted a decrease of the mean DLQI score from 9.9 at baseline to 2.4 after treatment. In a Canadian group of 146 patients with PAH the mean DLQI score decreased from 10.6 at baseline to 1.7 after 4 weeks.[6] Apart from investigation in patients with the most frequent types of PFH,[9,68–71] significant reductions of mean DLQI scores were also found after BoNT/A treatment of compensatory hyperhidrosis[13] and after botulinum neurotoxin type B treatment of primary craniofacial hyperhidrosis.[72] More rarely, DLQI assessment was also used in patients subjected to surgery[63,73,74] or treatment with oral anticholinergics.[10,14] In 51 patients the median DLQI score decreased from 12 before suction curettage to 4 at 9 months after surgery.[73] Improvement of the score was noted in almost two-thirds of patients. In 339 subjects treated with oral methantheline bromide or placebo, the mean DLQI score decreased from 16.4 at baseline to 9.7 after 4 weeks in the verum group, compared with 17 to 12.2 in the placebo group.[10]

A comparative literature analysis revealed that QoL impairment associated with PFH often equaled or exceeded that of severe dermatologic diseases such as atopic dermatitis, contact dermatitis, and psoriasis.[3]

Skindex

Skindex is another validated, self-administered instrument for measurement of the effects of skin disease on patients' QoL.[75] The questionnaire has 61 items on 8 scales, namely cognitive effects, social effects, depression, fear, embarrassment, anger, physical discomfort, and physical limitations. Item responses are standardized from 0 (no effect) to 100 (maximal effect). Skindex has been applied once to patients with PFH.[76] The mean score averaged 24.4 with slightly higher values in patients with axillary conditions than palmar conditions (25.1 and 23.7, respectively), reflecting considerable QoL impairment.

GENERAL ASSESSMENT OF QoL
Short Form Health Survey (36 Item and 12 Item)

The 36-item Short Form Health Survey (SF-36) and an abbreviated variant of it, the 12-item Short Form Health Survey (SF-12), are valid and reliable patient-reported tools widely used for evaluation of the health-related QoL of an individual.[77] The

SF-36 consists of multiple-choice questions on 8 health domains (vitality, physical functioning, bodily pain, general health perceptions, physical role functioning, emotional role functioning, social role functioning, mental health). Answers are transformed into scales and 2 main summaries, the Physical Component Summary (PCS) score and the Mental Component Summary (MCS) score. These norm-based scores range from 0 to 100 points with 50 points being the average Unites States score and with 10 points representing 1 standard deviation. The lower the score, the higher the disability.

Sayeed and colleagues[78] were the first to use the SF-36 tool to assess the QoL status before and after ETS in a small number of patients with upper limb hyperhidrosis. Since then, the SF-36 has emerged as the favored instrument in the assessment of general QoL in patients with PFH. Pretreatment SF-36 scores often showed lower than normal mental and physical health dimensions that improved after ETS surgery.[29,74,79–84] Strongest effects were mostly seen in social functioning and other scores of mental fitness. One study comparing SF-36 results in operated patients with those in healthy controls revealed no significant differences.[74] Only bodily pain and physical role domains decreased 1 month after ETS, because of the effects of the recent operation, but recovered shortly thereafter.[74,80] In a German study on 178 patients with PFH the SF-36 values for vitality, social fitness, and psychological fitness showed a tendency to smaller values in patients with postoperative compensatory sweating, but did not reach statistical relevance.[82] Lee and colleagues[31] observed increases in SF-36 scores in patients with PFH treated with oral glycopyrrolate.

In our study on 345 subjects with PFH the compressed SF-12 version of the questionnaire was used.[3] Compared with healthy controls, patients with hyperhidrosis had lower mean scores indicating poorer health status on both the MCS score (44.4 vs 50.8) and the PCS score (52.9 vs 54.9). In 240 patients with PAH treated with BoNT/A, the mean PCS score significantly improved from baseline by 0.9 points and the mean MCS score by 1.7 points.[40] Measures of SF-12 in 51 patients with various types of PFH showed significant mean increases 1 month after ETS in both PCS score (51.45 before ETS vs 54.25 after ETS) and MCS score (49.08 before ETS vs 53.88 after ETS).[84]

Other Instruments

On rare occasions, other instruments than the SF-36/SF-12 were used to rate the QoL impairment in patients with hyperhidrosis. Cinà and Clase[85] administered the Illness Intrusiveness Ratings Scale (IIRS) by electronic mail to patients with PFH, and 68 people responded on 2 occasions 4 weeks apart. The IIRS measures the extent to which a disease, its treatment, or both interfere with activities across 13 life domains considered important to QoL on a 7-point Likert scale. Scores were lower in participants who previously had surgery for hyperhidrosis, compared with those who had not, and improved dramatically in 4 patients who underwent surgery during the course of the study.[85]

The Nottingham Health Profile (NHP) contains 38 items dealing with the 6 health domains of pain, energy, sleep, mobility, emotional reaction, and social isolation. Ambrogi and colleagues[29] used it in patients with PPH for comparison of ETS and BoNT/A injections at different time points after treatment and noted the same trend for both the NHP and the simultaneously applied SF-36.

The Everyday Life Questionnaire (EDLQ) was used in 30 patients with PPH before and 6 months after ETS.[86] The instrument comprises 42 questions about physical, emotional, social, and functional components of QoL as well as joy of life and patient satisfaction with medical care. Poor preoperative QoL was a significant predictor of postoperative improvement across all dimensions covered by the questionnaire.

ASSESSMENT OF SPECIAL IMPAIRMENTS

Anxiety, depression, and social phobia profiles were repeatedly assessed in patients with hyperhidrosis.[31,49,76,84,87] Weber and colleagues[76] applied the State-Trait Anxiety Inventory G Form X2 (STAI), the Social Phobia Scale (SPS), the Symptom Checklist 90R (SCL-90-R) of Derogatis, and the Hospital Anxiety and Depression Scale (HADS-D) to 70 patients with different types of PFH. Only the mean value for SPS was slightly greater than the normal range, but values of all instruments significantly changed in the direction of normalization after BoNT/A treatment. Likewise, Ramos and colleagues[49] found that general state and trait anxiety levels in 158 patients with PPH and other types of PFH before ETS surgery were similar to those of the general population. However, when applying a self-designed anxiety-specific questionnaire inquiring typical incapacitating situations nearly half of the patients affirmed 9 or more of 14 questions. Items related to the hands and their use, to public situations, and relations with people of the opposite sex and strangers scored the highest. The investigators concluded that patients with PFH have a high degree of anxiety perceived as debilitating in daily life, which the STAI was unable to measure. In another 51 patients with PFH STAI rates bordered clinical significance, whereas depressive symptoms, as assessed by the Center for Epidemiologic Studies Depression Scale (CES-D), were not altered.[84] However, rates of both anxiety and depression were decreased 1 month after ETS. Beck Depression Inventory (BDI), Beck Anxiety Inventory (BAI), and the Autonomic Nervous System (ANS) scale were used in 2 studies on the effect of glycopyrrolate.[31,87] Only declines in the BAI score were noted in patients with PFH,[31] whereas decreases in both BAI score and BDI score occurred in patients with compensatory hyperhidrosis.[87]

A group of 50 patients with PFH recently scored significantly higher in 2 of 3 subscales of the Toronto Alexithymia Scale-20, a 20-item tool that measures features of alexithymia, denoting an insufficiency in identification and expression of emotions.[88] Values greater than normal were found in 45.6% of patients compared with 18.2% of control participants. Alexithymic individuals are less able to cope with stress and to communicate their feelings effectively, they tend to develop fewer close relationships, and have lesser social skills.[88] The same Turkish group of psychiatrists found significant differences in several scores of the Temperament and Character Inventory (TCI) between patients with PFH and controls.[89] The results indicate that patients with PFH might have less energy; might have a tendency to tiredness; and might be less able to tolerate, cope with, and recover from stress.

SUMMARY

Hyperhidrosis in general, and PFH in particular as the most important entity within its scope, are common conditions that are often detrimental to patients' social, psychological, professional, and physical well-being. Beyond objective measurement of increased sweat production and demarcation of affected sites and areas, the real impact of the disease can only be recognized by assessment of the reduction in QoL. Significant progress in treatment of PFH has been achieved by the introduction of botulinum toxin injections and the technical improvement of ETS, which is reflected in the intense QoL research since about the turn of the century. In the meanwhile, survey of QoL has become the most important outcome measure in patients with hyperhidrosis. The simplest tool for its rapid appraisal in daily routine is the HDSS. For more exact evaluation of QoL in clinical studies the use of a dermatology-specific instrument, such as the DLQI, and of a disease-specific instrument,

such as the HHIQ, are appropriate. The most suitable tool with a general section addressing limitations in social, psychological, private, and professional life as well as special sections identifying site-related problems probably has still to be developed. Use of a uniform questionnaire shared by dermatologists, thoracic surgeons, and other treating physicians is desirable, with a summed total score facilitating comparison. Additional use of instruments assessing general QoL issues and allowing the detection of typical disadvantages, side effects, and complications of different treatments before and during/after intervention also seems to be important. Otherwise, drawbacks such as expenditure of time in tap water iontophoresis, xerostomia caused by oral anticholinergics, and compensatory hyperhidrosis after ETS surgery may be missed.

REFERENCES

1. Adar R, Kurchin A, Zweig A, et al. Palmar hyperhidrosis and its surgical treatment: a report of 100 cases. Ann Surg 1977;186:34–41.
2. Mindus P. Livskvalitet och hyperhidros. Läkartidningen 1980;77:1999–2000.
3. Hamm H, Naumann MK, Kowalski JW, et al. Primary focal hyperhidrosis: disease characteristics and functional impairment. Dermatology 2006;212:343–53.
4. Walling HW. Primary hyperhidrosis increases the risk of cutaneous infection: a case-control study of 387 patients. J Am Acad Dermatol 2009;61:242–6.
5. Strutton DR, Kowalski JW, Glaser DA, et al. US prevalence of hyperhidrosis and impact on individuals with axillary hyperhidrosis: results from a national survey. J Am Acad Dermatol 2004;51:241–8.
6. Solish N, Benohanian A, Kowalski JW, et al. Prospective open-label study of botulinum toxin type A in patients with axillary hyperhidrosis: effects on functional impairment and quality of life. Dermatol Surg 2005;31:405–13.
7. Lowe NJ, Glaser DA, Eadie N, et al. Botulinum toxin type A in the treatment of primary axillary hyperhidrosis: a 52-week multicenter double-blind, randomized, placebo-controlled study of efficacy and safety. J Am Acad Dermatol 2007;56:604–11.
8. Yanagihara TK, Ibrahimiye A, Harris C, et al. Analysis of clamping versus cutting of T3 sympathetic nerve for severe palmar hyperhidrosis. J Thorac Cardiovasc Surg 2010;140:984–9.
9. Campanati A, Sandroni L, Gesuita R, et al. Treatment of focal idiopathic hyperhidrosis with botulinum toxin type A: clinical predictive factors of relapse-free survival. J Eur Acad Dermatol Venereol 2011;25:917–21.

10. Müller C, Berensmeier A, Hamm H, et al. Efficacy and safety of methantheline bromide (Vagantin(®)) in axillary and palmar hyperhidrosis: results from a multicenter, randomized, placebo-controlled trial. J Eur Acad Dermatol Venereol 2013;27: 1278–84.

11. Ibrahim O, Kakar R, Bolotin D, et al. The comparative effectiveness of suction-curettage and onabotulinumtoxin-A injections for the treatment of primary focal axillary hyperhidrosis: a randomized control trial. J Am Acad Dermatol 2013;69:88–95.

12. Solish N, Bertucci V, Dansereau A, et al. A comprehensive approach to the recognition, diagnosis, and severity-based treatment of focal hyperhidrosis: recommendations of the Canadian Hyperhidrosis Advisory Committee. Dermatol Surg 2007;33:908–23.

13. Kim WO, Kil HK, Yoon KB, et al. Botulinum toxin: a treatment for compensatory hyperhidrosis in the trunk. Dermatol Surg 2009;35:833–8.

14. Kim WO, Kil HK, Yoon KB, et al. Treatment of generalized hyperhidrosis with oxybutynin in postmenopausal patients. Acta Derm Venereol 2010; 90:291–3.

15. Kwong KF, Cooper LB, Bennett LA, et al. Clinical experience in 397 consecutive thoracoscopic sympathectomies. Ann Thorac Surg 2005;80:1063–6.

16. Kwong KF, Hobbs JL, Cooper LB, et al. Stratified analysis of clinical outcomes in thoracoscopic sympathicotomy for hyperhidrosis. Ann Thorac Surg 2008;85:390–3.

17. Amir M, Arish A, Weinstein Y, et al. Impairment in quality of life among patients seeking surgery for hyperhidrosis (excessive sweating): preliminary results. Isr J Psychiatry Relat Sci 2000;37:25–31.

18. De Campos JR, Kauffman P, Werebe Ede C, et al. Quality of life, before and after thoracic sympathectomy: report on 378 operated patients. Ann Thorac Surg 2003;76:886–91.

19. Yazbek G, Wolosker N, de Campos JR, et al. Palmar hyperhidrosis – which is the best level of denervation using video-assisted thoracoscopic sympathectomy: T2 or T3 ganglion? J Vasc Surg 2005;42:281–5.

20. Munia MA, Wolosker N, Kaufmann P, et al. Sustained benefit lasting one year from T4 instead of T3-T4 sympathectomy for isolated axillary hyperhidrosis. Clinics (Sao Paulo) 2008;63:771–4.

21. Wolosker N, Yazbek G, Ishy A, et al. Is sympathectomy at T4 level better than at T3 level for treating palmar hyperhidrosis? J Laparoendosc Adv Surg Tech A 2008;18:102–6.

22. Yazbek G, Wolosker N, Kauffman P, et al. Twenty months of evolution following sympathectomy on patients with palmar hyperhidrosis: sympathectomy at the T3 level is better than at the T2 level. Clinics (Sao Paulo) 2009;64:743–9.

23. Wolosker N, Munia MA, Kauffman P, et al. Is gender a predictive factor for satisfaction among patients undergoing sympathectomy to treat palmar hyperhidrosis? Clinics (Sao Paulo) 2010;65:583–6.

24. Wolosker N, Yazbek G, de Campos JR, et al. Quality of life before surgery is a predictive factor for satisfaction among patients undergoing sympathectomy to treat hyperhidrosis. J Vasc Surg 2010;51:1190–4.

25. Ishy A, de Campos JR, Wolosker N, et al. Objective evaluation of patients with palmar hyperhidrosis submitted to two levels of sympathectomy: T3 and T4. Interact Cardiovasc Thorac Surg 2011;12:545–8.

26. Wolosker N, de Campos JR, Kauffman P, et al. Evaluation of quality of life over time among 453 patients with hyperhidrosis submitted to endoscopic thoracic sympathectomy. J Vasc Surg 2012;55:154–6.

27. Neves S, Uchoa PC, Wolosker N, et al. Long-term comparison of video-assisted thoracic sympathectomy and clinical observation for the treatment of palmar hyperhidrosis in children younger than 14. Pediatr Dermatol 2012;29:575–9.

28. Loureiro Mde P, de Campos JR, Kauffman P, et al. Endoscopic lumbar sympathectomy for women: effect on compensatory sweat. Clinics (Sao Paulo) 2008;63:189–96.

29. Ambrogi V, Campione E, Mineo D, et al. Bilateral thoracoscopic T2 to T3 sympathectomy versus botulinum injection in palmar hyperhidrosis. Ann Thorac Surg 2009;88:238–45.

30. Wang FG, Chen YB, Yang WT, et al. Comparison of compensatory sweating and quality of life following thoracic sympathetic block for palmar hyperhidrosis: electrocautery hook versus titanium clip. Chin Med J (Engl) 2011;124:3495–8.

31. Lee HH, Kim do W, Kim do W, et al. Efficacy of glycopyrrolate in primary hyperhidrosis patients. Korean J Pain 2012;25:28–32.

32. Panhofer P, Gleiss A, Eilenberg WH, et al. Long-term outcomes after endothoracic sympathetic block at the T4 ganglion for upper limb hyperhidrosis. Br J Surg 2013;100:1471–7.

33. Wolosker N, de Campos JR, Kauffman P, et al. An alternative to treat palmar hyperhidrosis: use of oxybutynin. Clin Auton Res 2011;21:389–93.

34. Wolosker N, de Campos JR, Kauffman P, et al. The use of oxybutynin for treating axillary hyperhidrosis. Ann Vasc Surg 2011;25:1057–62.

35. Wolosker N, de Campos JR, Kauffman P, et al. A randomized placebo-controlled trial of oxybutynin for the initial treatment of palmar and axillary hyperhidrosis. J Vasc Surg 2012;55:1696–700.

36. Wolosker N, Krutman M, Campdell TP, et al. Oxybutynin treatment for hyperhidrosis: a comparative analysis between genders. Einstein (Sao Paulo) 2012;10:405–8.

37. Wolosker N, Krutman M, Kauffman P, et al. Effectiveness of oxybutynin for treatment of hyperhidrosis in overweight and obese patients. Rev Assoc Med Bras 2013;59:143–7.

38. Wolosker N, Schvartsman C, Krutman M, et al. Efficacy and quality of life outcomes of oxybutynin for treating palmar hyperhidrosis in children younger than 14 years old. Pediatr Dermatol 2014; 31:48–53.

39. Teale C, Roberts G. Development, validity, and reliability of the Hyperhidrosis Impact Questionnaire (HHIQ) (abstract). Qual Life Res 2002;11:702.

40. Naumann MK, Hamm H, Lowe NJ, et al. Effect of botulinum toxin type A on quality of life measures in patients with excessive axillary sweating: a randomized controlled trial. Br J Dermatol 2002;147: 1218–26.

41. Naumann M, Lowe NJ, Kumar CR, et al. Botulinum toxin type A is a safe and effective treatment for axillary hyperhidrosis over 16 months: a prospective study. Arch Dermatol 2003;139:731–6.

42. Keller S, Sekons D, Scher H, et al. A novel scale for assessing quality of life following bilateral endoscopic thoracic sympathectomy for palmar and plantar hyperhidrosis. In: Abstract Book of the 4th International Symposium on Sympathetic Surgery. Abstract O–22. Tampere (Finland), June 28–30, 2001.

43. Neumayer C, Zacherl J, Holak G, et al. Limited endoscopic thoracic sympathetic block for hyperhidrosis of the upper limb: reduction of compensatory sweating by clipping T4. Surg Endosc 2004; 18:152–6.

44. Neumayer C, Panhofer P, Zacherl J, et al. Effect of endoscopic thoracic sympathetic block on plantar hyperhidrosis. Arch Surg 2005;140:676–80.

45. Panhofer P, Zacherl J, Jakesz R, et al. Improved quality of life after sympathetic block for upper limb hyperhidrosis. Br J Surg 2006;93:582–6.

46. Ghisletta N, Habicht J, Stulz P. Video-assisted thoracosopic sympathectomy: spectrum of indications and our own results (1995-1997). Schweiz Med Wochenschr 1999;129:985–92.

47. Kuo CH, Yen M, Lin PC. Developing an instrument to measure quality of life of patients with hyperhidrosis. J Nurs Res 2004;12:21–30.

48. Loscertales J, Arroyo Tristán A, Congregado Loscertales M, et al. Thoracoscopic sympathectomy for palmar hyperhidrosis. Immediate results and postoperative quality of life. Arch Bronconeumol 2004;40:67–71.

49. Ramos R, Moya J, Turón V, et al. [Primary hyperhidrosis and anxiety: a prospective preoperative survey of 158 patients]. Arch Bronconeumol 2005;41:88–92.

50. Cinà CS, Cinà MM, Clase CM. Endoscopic thoracic sympathectomy for hyperhidrosis: technique and results. J Minim Access Surg 2007;3:132–40.

51. Ottomann C, Blazek J, Hartmann B, et al. Liposuction curettage versus Botox for axillary hyperhidrosis. A prospective study of the quality of life. Chirurg 2007;78:356–61.

52. Jaffer U, Weedon K, Cameron AE. Factors affecting outcome following endoscopic thoracic sympathectomy. Br J Surg 2007;94:1108–12.

53. Boley TM, Belangee KN, Markwell S, et al. The effect of thoracoscopic sympathectomy on quality of life and symptom management of hyperhidrosis. J Am Coll Surg 2007;204:435–8.

54. Jeganathan R, Jordan S, Jones M, et al. Bilateral thoracoscopic sympathectomy: results and long-term follow-up. Interact Cardiovasc Thorac Surg 2008;7:67–70.

55. Libson S, Kirshtein B, Mizrahi S, et al. Evaluation of compensatory sweating after bilateral thoracoscopic sympathectomy for palmar hyperhidrosis. Surg Laparosc Endosc Percutan Tech 2007;17: 511–3.

56. Steiner Z, Cohen Z, Kleiner O, et al. Do children tolerate thoracoscopic sympathectomy better than adults? Pediatr Surg Int 2008;24:343–7.

57. Hartl DM, Julieron M, LeRidant AM, et al. Botulinum toxin A for quality of life improvement in post-parotidectomy gustatory sweating (Frey's syndrome). J Laryngol Otol 2008;122:1100–4.

58. Coutinho dos Santos LH, Gomes AM, Giraldi S, et al. Palmar hyperhidrosis: long-term follow-up of nine children and adolescents treated with botulinum toxin type A. Pediatr Dermatol 2009;26: 439–44.

59. Bachmann K, Standl N, Kaifi J, et al. Thoracoscopic sympathectomy for palmar and axillary hyperhidrosis: four-year outcome and quality of life after bilateral 5-mm dual port approach. Surg Endosc 2009;23:1587–93.

60. Cardoso PO, Rodrigues KC, Mendes KM, et al. Evaluation of patients submitted to surgical treatment for palmar hyperhidrosis with regard to the quality of life and to the appearance of compensatory hyperhidrosis. Rev Col Bras Cir 2009;36:14–8.

61. Prasad A, Ali M, Kaul S. Endoscopic thoracic sympathectomy for primary palmar hyperidrosis. Surg Endosc 2010;24:1952–7.

62. Marcella S, Goodman G, Cumming S, et al. Thirty-five units of botulinum toxin type A for treatment of axillary hyperhidrosis in female patients. Australas J Dermatol 2011;52:123–6.

63. Garcia Franco CE, Perez-Cajaraville J, Guillen-Grima F, et al. Prospective study of percutaneous radiofrequency sympathicolysis in severe hyperhidrosis and facial blushing: efficacy and safety findings. Eur J Cardiothorac Surg 2011;40:e146–51.

64. Vanderhelst E, De Keukeleire T, Verbanck S, et al. Quality of life and patient satisfaction after video-assisted thoracic sympathicolysis for essential

hyperhidrosis: a follow-up of 138 patients. J Laparoendosc Adv Surg Tech A 2011;21:905–9.

65. Zhu LH, Du Q, Chen L, et al. One-year follow-up period after transumbilical thoracic sympathectomy for hyperhidrosis: outcomes and consequences. J Thorac Cardiovasc Surg 2014;147: 25–8.

66. Finlay AY, Khan GK. Dermatology Life Quality Index (DLQI): a simple practical measure for routine clinical use. Clin Exp Dermatol 1994;19:210–6.

67. Swartling C, Naver H, Lindberg M. Botulinum A toxin improves life quality in severe primary focal hyperhidrosis. Eur J Neurol 2001;8:247–52.

68. Tan SR, Solish N. Long-term efficacy and quality of life in the treatment of focal hyperhidrosis with botulinum toxin A. Dermatol Surg 2002;28:495–9.

69. Campanati A, Penna L, Guzzo T, et al. Quality-of-life assessment in patients with hyperhidrosis before and after treatment with botulinum toxin: results of an open-label study. Clin Ther 2003;25: 298–308.

70. Campanati A, Bernardini ML, Gesuita R, et al. Plantar focal idiopathic hyperhidrosis and botulinum toxin: a pilot study. Eur J Dermatol 2007;17: 52–4.

71. Rosell K, Hymnelius K, Swartling C. Botulinum toxin type A and B improve quality of life in patients with axillary and palmar hyperhidrosis. Acta Derm Venereol 2013;93:335–9.

72. Karlqvist M, Rosell K, Rystedt A, et al. Botulinum toxin B in the treatment of craniofacial hyperhidrosis. J Eur Acad Dermatol Venereol 2013. http://dx.doi.org/10.1111/jdv.12278. [Epub ahead of print].

73. Bechara FG, Gambichler T, Bader A, et al. Assessment of quality of life in patients with primary axillary hyperhidrosis before and after suction-curettage. J Am Acad Dermatol 2007;57:207–12.

74. Tetteh HA, Groth SS, Kast T, et al. Primary palmoplantar hyperhidrosis and thoracoscopic sympathectomy: a new objective assessment method. Ann Thorac Surg 2009;87:267–74.

75. Chren MM, Lasek RJ, Quinn LM, et al. Skindex, a quality-of-life measure for patients with skin disease: reliability, validity, and responsiveness. J Invest Dermatol 1996;107:707–13.

76. Weber A, Heger S, Sinkgraven R, et al. Psychosocial aspects of patients with focal hyperhidrosis. Marked reduction of social phobia, anxiety and depression and increased quality of life after treatment with botulinum toxin A. Br J Dermatol 2005; 152:342–5.

77. Ware JE Jr, Sherbourne CD. The MOS 36-item short-form health survey (SF-36). I. Conceptual framework and item selection. Med Care 1992;30: 473–83.

78. Sayeed RA, Nyamekye I, Ghauri AS, et al. Quality of life after transthoracic endoscopic sympathectomy for upper limb hyperhidrosis. Eur J Surg Suppl 1998;(580):39–42.

79. Young O, Neary P, Keaveny TV, et al. Evaluation of the impact of transthoracic endoscopic sympathectomy on patients with palmar hyperhydrosis. Eur J Vasc Endovasc Surg 2003;26:673–6.

80. Kumagai K, Kawase H, Kawanishi M. Health-related quality of life after thoracoscopic sympathectomy for palmar hyperhidrosis. Ann Thorac Surg 2005;80:461–6.

81. Elia S, Guggino G, Mineo D, et al. Awake one stage bilateral thoracoscopic sympathectomy for palmar hyperhidrosis: a safe outpatient procedure. Eur J Cardiothorac Surg 2005;28:312–7.

82. Schmidt J, Bechara FG, Altmeyer P, et al. Endoscopic thoracic sympathectomy for severe hyperhidrosis: impact of restrictive denervation on compensatory sweating. Ann Thorac Surg 2006; 81:1048–55.

83. Rodríguez PM, Freixinet JL, Hussein M, et al. Side effects, complications and outcome of thoracoscopic sympathectomy for palmar and axillary hyperhidrosis in 406 patients. Eur J Cardiothorac Surg 2008;34:514–9.

84. Vazquez LD, Staples NL, Sears SF, et al. Psychosocial functioning of patients after endoscopic thoracic sympathectomy. Eur J Cardiothorac Surg 2011;39:1018–21.

85. Cinà CS, Clase CM. The Illness Intrusiveness Rating Scale: a measure of severity in individuals with hyperhidrosis. Qual Life Res 1999;8:693–8.

86. Koskinen LO, Blomstedt P, Sjöberg RL. Predicting improvement after surgery for palmar hyperhidrosis. Acta Neurol Scand 2012;126:324–8.

87. Gong TK, Kim do W. Effectiveness of oral glycopyrrolate use in compensatory hyperhidrosis patients. Korean J Pain 2013;26:89–93.

88. Ak M, Dinçer D, Haciomeroglu B, et al. The evaluation of primary idiopathic focal hyperhidrosis patients in terms of alexithymia. J Health Psychol 2013;18:704–10.

89. Ak M, Dincer D, Haciomeroglu B, et al. Temperament and character properties of primary focal hyperhidrosis patients. Health Qual Life Outcomes 2013;11:5.

Special Considerations for Children with Hyperhidrosis

Benjamin R. Bohaty, MD[a], Adelaide A. Hebert, MD[a,b],*

KEYWORDS

- Hyperhidrosis • Iontophoresis • Botulinum toxin • Pediatric population

KEY POINTS

- Primary hyperhidrosis has traditionally been considered a medical and psychosocial problem for adult patients, with estimates suggesting that 1.6% of adolescents and 0.6% of prepubertal children are affected by this condition.
- A thorough history and physical examination should be performed to help rule out an underlying causation for secondary hyperhidrosis before initiating treatment.
- Quality of life in the pediatric population can be significantly improved by early diagnosis and therapy.
- Many therapeutic options for primary pediatric hyperhidrosis exist including topical and systemic therapies, iontophoresis, and botulinum toxin injections.

INTRODUCTION

Hyperhidrosis is a condition characterized by excess sweat production affecting children and adults. Primary focal hyperhidrosis is currently considered to be idiopathic, affecting areas of the body including the axillae, palms, soles, and face. Primary hyperhidrosis is believed to occur as a result of a hyperactive sympathetic nervous system.[1] Secondary hyperhidrosis, which usually results from an underlying condition, can present in a focal or generalized pattern. A thorough history and physical examination can help to rule out an underlying causation for secondary hyperhidrosis. The prevalence of hyperhidrosis in the United States has been estimated to be 2.9%, with an average age of onset of 14 to 25 years.[2–4] Primary hyperhidrosis has traditionally been considered a problem for adults, but estimates show that 1.6% of adolescents and 0.6% of prepubertal children are affected.[2] The primary locations of involvement in pediatric subjects include the palmoplantar and axillary areas.[4,5]

Psychological and social development and well-being are often affected, impacting patient quality of life, which may in turn lead to profound emotional and social distress.[2,5,6] Pediatric subjects with hyperhidrosis can have difficulties handing a writing utensil, keeping papers dry, gripping the handlebar of a bicycle, manipulating a computer mouse, and using a video game controller.[6] Quality of life can be significantly improved by early diagnosis and therapy; however, underdiagnosis and lack of

Funding Sources/Conflict of Interest: Allergan (note: all research funds were paid to The University of Texas Medical School - Houston, Houston, Texas; Protocol Number 191622-075-00, Allergan, 2005 – 2007) (A.A. Hebert); No conflicts to report (B.R. Bohaty).
[a] Department of Dermatology, The University of Texas Health Science Center at Houston, 6655 Travis Street, Suite 980, Houston, TX 77030, USA; [b] Department of Pediatrics, The University of Texas Health Science Center at Houston, Houston, TX, USA
* Corresponding author. Department of Dermatology, The University of Texas Health Science Center at Houston, 6655 Travis Street, Suite 980, Houston, TX 77030.
E-mail address: Adelaide.a.hebert@uth.tmc.edu

Dermatol Clin 32 (2014) 477–484
http://dx.doi.org/10.1016/j.det.2014.06.005
0733-8635/14/$ – see front matter © 2014 Elsevier Inc. All rights reserved.

knowledge regarding therapeutic options has hindered maximization of therapy in the pediatric population.[7] The medical community is not solely to blame for failure to provide or delayed treatment options. In a survey performed by Strutton and coworkers[2] only 38% of patients with hyperhidrosis had sought medical assistance for their excessive sweating. The risk for concomitant cutaneous disease (eg, verruca vulgaris, dermatophytosis) is increased for patients with hyperhidrosis.[8] This article explores the available therapeutic options for pediatric hyperhidrosis, and expands awareness of this frequently underrecognized medical condition.

TOPICAL THERAPY

Treatment options for hyperhidrosis in the pediatric population are somewhat limited.[7,9] Topical medications are often the first-line therapy and frequently include aluminum salts, which are found in over-the-counter and prescription antiperspirants. Aluminum chloride hexahydrate is the active ingredient found in prescription preparations, whereas a partially neutralized version is used in nonprescription compounds.[10] Topical aluminum chloride preparations are thought to mechanically obstruct eccrine sweat gland pores and lead to atrophy of the secretory cells.[11] Aluminum chloride hexahydrate 20% to 25% preparations in alcohol have been found to be effective first-line treatments for axillary hyperhidrosis.[12,13] Treatment regimen during one study consisted of patients applying the solution nightly for 1 week and then as needed, with most patients needing to reapply only once every 7 to 21 days to maintain adequate control. The only side effect reported during this study was irritation at the application site, which responded to treatment with 1% hydrocortisone for most that were affected.[13] Aluminum chloride therapy is less effective at treating palmar hyperhidrosis. A study published in 1990 by Goh[14] found that palmar hyperhidrosis was reduced within 48 hours of treatment with topical aluminum chloride 20%; however, this efficacy was lost 2 days after cessation of treatment. Local irritation and posttreatment pruritus and burning were the major limitations for this treatment modality.

A newer formulation of aluminum chloride hexahydrate using a hydroalcoholic gel base containing 4% salicylic acid was evaluated in a study of 238 patients with palmoplantar and axillary hyperhidrosis. This base was chosen to enhance absorption and minimize the irritant side effects associated with the traditional alcohol bases. Patients with palmar, plantar, and axillary disease had excellent-to-good response rates with values of 60%, 84%,

and 94%, respectively. Nonresponders and those with adverse reactions to earlier aluminum chloride preparations demonstrated better tolerance and control of disease with this new hydrogel compound.[15]

Other topical applications, such as astringents (eg, formaldehyde, glutaraldehyde, tannic acid), have shown efficacy in the treatment of hyperhidrosis, but their use is limited because of their propensity to cause staining of the skin and sensitization reactions.[16]

The efficacy and safety of topical treatments has rarely been studied in the pediatric population. However, topical aluminum chloride preparations remain popular among pediatric prescribers because of their relatively benign safety profile and ease of application. Downsides to treatment with topical products include the need for frequent reapplication to maintain efficacy, and local side effects including burning and pruritus. In addition, topical therapy is not effective for all those affected by hyperhidrosis, leaving some to explore other treatment options.

ANTICHOLINERGICS

Anticholinergic medications have been available for many decades and have widely been used to help minimize secretions perioperatively, and to decrease salivation in pediatric patients with neurologic conditions.[17,18] The ability of anticholinergic medications to improve hyperhidrosis was inadvertently revealed when patients given preparations from atropine plants developed a decrease in sweat production.[19] Anticholinergic medications competitively antagonize the muscarinic acetylcholine receptors, which are a prominent component of glandular tissue.[20,21]

A few case reports have demonstrated efficacy of topical anticholinergic preparations in such conditions as craniofacial hyperhidrosis and diabetic gustatory sweating. However, randomized controlled trials are needed to accurately determine efficacy and safety.[10,22–24]

Oral anticholinergic use in the treatment of hyperhidrosis is becoming increasingly more common, and agents include such drugs as glycopyrrolate and propantheline bromide. Annual treatment with generic oral glycopyrrolate at a dosage of 2 mg/day has been estimated to cost $756 per year, which is a fraction of the cost for treatment with botulinum toxin injections.[5] Side effects of anticholinergic medications can be limiting at the doses required for efficacy and include xerostomia most frequently, and blurred vision, tachycardia, urinary hesitancy, and constipation.[16,25] To help determine the efficacy of oral glycopyrrolate in the treatment of hyperhidrosis, Bajaj and Langtry[21] conducted a retrospective analysis of 24 adult subjects ages 19 to 62 that were treated with oral glycopyrrolate. This study found that 79% of those treated with glycopyrrolate had a positive response; however, the side effects limited further treatment of some of the participating individuals.[21]

More recently, Paller and coworkers[5] conducted a retrospective analysis of 31 pediatric patients with primary focal hyperhidrosis who were treated with a mean dosage of 2 mg of oral glycopyrrolate daily for an average of 2.1 years. The analysis demonstrated a positive response in 90% of those treated, which was major in 71% of responders. Side effects were experienced by 29% of the treated pediatric subjects, the most common of which included xerostomia (26%) and xerophthalmia (10%). These side effects were noted to be dose-related. The authors concluded that oral glycopyrrolate is an inexpensive, well-tolerated, and painless second-line treatment of pediatric subjects with primary focal hyperhidrosis.[5]

Another institutional review by Kumar and coworkers[26] looked at 12 children with severe, refractory hyperhidrosis treated with oral glycopyrrolate from July 2009 to January 2012. The average length of therapy was 18 months and the most common dosing regimen was 1 mg/day. Eleven (92%) of 12 patients noted improvement, and 9 (75%) of 12 would recommend oral glycopyrrolate to a friend. Seven patients noted side effects, none of which were severe. Dry mouth was the most common side effect and was reported in 50% of those treated (N = 6). Other side effects included constipation (N = 1), dizziness (N = 1), and facial swelling (N = 1). This retrospective analysis provides additional support that oral glycopyrrolate is a safe and effective treatment in children with hyperhidrosis.

A recent retrospective study of pediatric patients aged 10 to 18 years found that subjects with hyperhidrosis who were prescribed glycopyrrolate had on average a three-point improvement (on a five-point scale) in sweating reduction. Most subjects took the medication twice daily to achieve ideal control of sweating. Despite side effects, which included dry mouth (82%), constipation (55%), dry eyes (16%), palpitations (36%), and urinary retention (18%), glycopyrrolate was the preferred treatment of this cohort of patients, because of the rapid onset of action and efficacy of the medication. Additionally, these pediatric patients were remarkably compliant with the glycopyrrolate treatment schedule as prescribed. Half the patients reported refilling their prescription within 1 week of running out of pills. Reasons cited for not taking glycopyrrolate on a regular basis by this pediatric population included being bothered by side effects (62%), lack of efficacy (26%), expense of the medication (15%), and forgetting to take the medication (16%). Of the patients included, 22% were male and 7% were female. Seventy-nine percent of the patients reported their ethnicity to be white, 11% were Hispanic, 7% were Asian, and 3% were of African American descent. Of the patients who participated in the study, 40% had generalized hyperhidrosis, 7% had axillary hyperhidrosis, 41% had palmoplantar hyperhidrosis, 5% had facial hyperhidrosis, and 7% had plantar hyperhidrosis. The duration of hyperhidrosis diagnosis at the time of survey completion was greater than 8 years for 15%, 5 to 8 years for 25%, 1 to 4 years for 48%, and less than 6 months for 12% of responders.[27]

IONTOPHORESIS

Beginning in the 1930s, electric current has been used to introduce ions into skin in a process known as iontophoresis. For decades this process had been conducted at health care facilities under the supervision of medical staff, but eventually made its way into the home in the year 1984.[28] Unadulterated tap water is the most common medium used to conduct the electric current into the cutaneous tissues. However, anticholinergic drugs can also be added to enhance efficacy at the cost of increasing the risk of systemic adverse effects, such as dry or sore throat.[29]

Despite its many years of effective use, the mechanism of action of iontophoresis remains under debate. Theories for the mechanism range from increased keratinization and plugging of eccrine ducts to alterations in electrochemical signaling, which may prevent the initial stimulus that causes the eccrine gland to perspire. A selective targeting of the eccrine glands because of their locally increased electrolyte concentration has also been proposed, which may lead to protein coagulation and a loss of eccrine function.[29,30]

Iontophoresis has proved effective in the treatment of hyperhidrosis involving the palms and soles. However, treatment of other affected areas, such as the axillae, remains impractical because of the challenges of delivering the iontophoresis to the axillae. The limitations of iontophoresis include the necessity for frequent retreatment to maintain efficacy (which is lost a few weeks after cessation of treatment), and the risk of local and systemic side effects.[16] Local side effects are mild and include erythema, stinging, vesiculation, and papulation at the sites of treatment.

Although iontophoresis has not been studied in the pediatric population specifically, pediatric subjects have been included as members of larger cohorts in more than one study. A single-blind prospective study by Dolianitis and coworkers[29] sought to determine the efficacy of iontophoresis with glycopyrrolate as compared with iontophoresis with tap water alone in 20 subjects ranging in age from 12 to 50 years with moderate to severe palmoplantar hyperhidrosis. Iontophoresis containing glycopyrrolate 0.05% in solution was found to have superior efficacy to iontophoresis with tap water alone. This efficacy was further enhanced and prolonged when treatment was bilateral as opposed to unilateral leading the investigators to hypothesize that a systemic action of glycopyrrolate was contributing to the local effects.[29]

A younger population of patients with hyperhidrosis aged 8 to 32 years was evaluated in a different study that also sought to evaluate the efficacy of iontophoresis. A total of 112 patients were treated and 81.2% were satisfied following the series of eight treatment sessions. More than half the subjects treated noted an improvement in plantar sweating following treatment, even though only the palms were subjected to iontophoresis during the study.[30] This evidence further supports a plausible systemic efficacy for iontophoresis following local treatment alone.

BOTULINUM TOXIN

The anaerobic bacterium known as *Clostridium botulinum* is responsible for the production of botulinum toxins. Seven distinct serotypes classified by their antigenic differences work by cleaving proteins necessary for fusion of acetylcholine vesicles with the presynaptic membrane thus inhibiting acetylcholine release from the sympathetic cholinergic nerve terminals. Therefore, a decrease in sweat production is achieved through intradermal botulinum toxin injection, which inhibits neurotransmission by affecting the nerve terminals that innervate sweat glands. The two serotypes of botulinum toxin used most commonly in the clinical realm are toxins A and B, which cleave receptor proteins SNAP-25 and synaptobrevin, respectively. Both have been found to have similar efficacy for the treatment of axillary hyperhidrosis. However, botulinum toxin A had a lower incidence of autonomic side effects and pain at the injection site, which likely contributed to its preferential use by most clinicians.[31,32] Botulinum toxin A (Botox; Allergan, Irvine, CA) was approved by the Food and Drug Administration (FDA) in 2004 for the treatment of severe primary axillary hyperhidrosis in adults. Two newer class A botulinum toxins (Dysport; Ipsen Biopharm, Wrexham, UK; Xeomin; Merz Pharmaceuticals Inc, Greensboro, NC) have

been approved by the FDA in 2009 and 2011, respectively, for the treatment of other conditions (eg, cervical dystonia) but have not yet received FDA approval for the treatment of hyperhidrosis. The FDA approved botulinum toxin B (Myobloc; Solstice Neurosciences, Malvern, PA) for the treatment of cervical dystonia only, thus leaving its use in the management of hyperhidrosis to be categorized as "off label."[10] A lack of FDA approval for the treatment of hyperhidrosis in children often forces affected individuals to pay out-of-pocket for treatment estimated to cost a minimum of $2400 annually.[5,6,9,33]

Injection Site Pain

Injection site pain is a major limiting factor for intradermal injections of botulinum toxin, although options exist to help minimize this pain. Application of topical anesthetics and cryotreatment before injection with botulinum toxin are only partially effective but may provide mild short-term relief. Dichlorotetrafluoroethane-containing refrigerant sprays have been shown to demonstrate some efficacy in reducing injection site discomfort.[34] One effective option for pain control is intravenous regional anesthesia via a procedure termed "Bier's block." This procedure may lack practicality in an outpatient dermatology office because it can lead to cardiovascular and central nervous system toxicity necessitating close cardiac monitoring throughout the procedure.[34] Management of palmar and/or plantar hyperhidrosis with digital block anesthesia at the wrists and/or ankles is a safe and effective option and can be performed in the outpatient setting. Nerve block at the median and ulnar nerve can lead to temporary weakness of the hand musculature postprocedure and paresthesias if the needle pierces the nerve during the anesthetizing process. General anesthesia in an operating room setting is arguably the most effective option to minimize pain during treatment; however, the increased cost to the patient and risks of general anesthesia should be weighed against the expected benefits.

Adverse Effects

Injection of botulinum toxin may lead to other adverse effects including bruising at the injection site, xerosis, and weakness of hand musculature that tends to be transient. Superficial injection of the toxin may minimize the risk for posttreatment muscle weakness.[34] In 2009, based on a safety evaluation of the botulinum toxin products, the FDA added a Boxed Warning to the prescribing information on this medication class to highlight that botulinum toxin may spread from the area of injection to produce symptoms consistent with botulism, such as muscle weakness, dysphonia, dysarthria, incontinence, trouble breathing, dysphagia, blurred vision, drooping eyelids, and death. Children treated for spasticity may receive several hundred units of botulinum toxin at a therapeutic session and have the potential for the greatest risk for these symptoms, but the symptomatology can also occur in adults. No definitive serious adverse event reports of distant spread of toxin effect have been associated with dermatologic use of botulinum toxin A at approved doses in children or adults.

Safety and Efficacy in Children

The safety and efficacy of botulinum toxin A for the treatment of severe axillary hyperhidrosis was first studied in adults. In a large multicenter 52-week, randomized, placebo-controlled trial in patients aged 18 to 75 with primary axillary hyperhidrosis, repeated botulinum toxin A injections were found to be safe and efficacious substantially reducing impairment in 75% of those treated at 1 month postinjection.[35] Data from this study, coupled with that from a later 3-year open-label extension of greater than 175 adult patients with primary axillary hyperhidrosis treated by intradermal injections of botulinum toxin, elucidated no serious adverse effects.[36]

The first report of botulinum toxin treatment of hyperhidrosis in the pediatric population arose in 2002 and described a 13-year-old girl who was treated for refractory hyperhidrosis of the palms.[37] Over a 2-year period she received a total of four rounds of injections that were successful in decreasing her palmar sweating, although she did experience an episode of transient muscle weakness of the hands lasting about 3 weeks. Since then, other case reports of successful treatment of refractory palmar hyperhidrosis in the pediatric population have been reported.[34] Not until 2005 were injections for hyperhidrosis of the axillae reported in the pediatric literature. A 14-year-old girl with severe refractory hyperhidrosis of the axillae leading to social distress and bad posture was treated with botulinum toxin A injections into each axilla. At follow-up 3 months posttreatment, she was noted to have a significant improvement in symptoms, including improved posture and social functioning.[38] Coutinho dos Santos and coworkers[6] conducted the largest case series to date that included a total of nine children or adolescents with palmar hyperhidrosis. All nine of the subjects that received botulinum type A injections demonstrated efficacy 1 month after one to four rounds of treatment. Although

botulinum toxin A has previously been used successfully and safely in the treatment of many other pediatric conditions (eg, cerebral palsy, torticollois, strabismus) randomized controlled trials in the treatment of primary pediatric hyperhidrosis are lacking, and more research is needed to definitively determine safety and efficacy.

SURGICAL TREATMENT

For patients with hyperhidrosis that is absolutely refractory to the less invasive treatments, surgical treatment may be a suitable option.

Liposuction

The least invasive of the surgical procedures includes liposuction of adipose tissue or curettage, which functions to remove the eccrine glands from the axillae, thus minimizing the sweat produced in that region over the long term. This procedure does not come without risks. Scarring, surgical site contractures, and infection have been noted; however, there is no risk for the compensatory sweating that can occur following more invasive surgical procedures, such as sympathectomy.[39]

Ultrasound

Another minimally invasive treatment of hyperhidrosis involves the use of the VASER System (Sound Surgical Technologies, Louisville, CO), which is a third-generation ultrasound system that has widely been used for body-contouring surgery. Treatment of the bilateral axillae takes approximately 1 hour and can be done as an outpatient with local anesthesia only. A prospective pilot-study published in 2009 investigated VASER efficacy in the treatment of 13 adult patients aged 25 to 52 years with significant axillary hyperhidrosis and/or bromidrosis that was refractory to other nonsurgical treatments. A significant reduction in sweat and odor and no recurrence of significant symptoms at 6 months was noted in 11 of 13 subjects who were treated. Two patients noted a decrease in sweat and odor, but the reduction was not as great as they had wished. Although no serious side effects were observed during this pilot study, three complications from the 26 axillae treated included one small seroma, one hyperpigmented area, and one blister (6 mm × 7 mm), all of which resolved spontaneously. Other potential side effects may include dysesthesia, transient or prolonged tissue swelling, bruising, infection, and hematoma formation.[40] Although this treatment option has not yet received FDA approval for the treatment of hyperhidrosis in children or adults, it seems to show promise as an emerging safe and effective minimally invasive surgical option for the treatment of refractory axillary hyperhidrosis.

Thoracic Sympathectomy

More invasive procedures for the treatment of focal hyperhidrosis involve destruction of the sympathetic chain, which in turn prevents neurotransmission to the cholinergic fibers that signal the onset of sweating. This destruction has traditionally been done with a more invasive method termed thoracic sympathectomy, and more recently replaced with less invasive procedures termed video-assisted thoracoscopic sympathectomy or endoscopic thoracic sympathectomy (ETS) that use smaller incisions and modern imaging techniques. Thoracic sympathectomy for the treatment of hyperhidrosis was first performed in Europe in the 1920s. Access to the thorax required division of one or more major muscles of the chest wall along with rib separation, which had the potential to cause significant pain and bone fractures in addition to the complications that are also seen with ETS.[39,41] This procedure is uncommonly performed in children today, having been widely replaced by more modern surgical techniques beginning as early as the 1940s.[5,42]

Video-Assisted Thoracoscopic Sympathectomy

Video-assisted thoracoscopic sympathectomy is now the most common technique used for the treatment of hyperhidrosis. After two to three incisions (typically no more than 1 cm) are made inferior to the axillae, the patient's lung is deflated, and a telescopic camera is introduced into the thoracic cavity. After the sympathetic chain is located, specific ganglia (ranging from T2 to T4) are destroyed that correlate with the areas of intended treatment effect (palmar vs axillary). Electrocautery and laser are commonly used for this destructive process.[43] Although the video-assisted procedures result in shorter recovery times, decrease postoperative pain, and minimize surgical site scarring, they are not without serious complications. Infection, compensatory sweating in surrounding areas, Horner syndrome, and several lung complications (eg, pneumothorax, hemothorax, atelectasis, subcutaneous emphysema) can occur.[39,41] Postsurgical compensatory hyperhidrosis ranging from mild to severe is common (>70%) and seems to better tolerated in children in turn leading to higher postoperative satisfaction according to at least one study.[44] Severe compensatory hyperhidrosis has been reported to be 40% in patients following ETS[10]; however, this risk can be lowered with a slightly different procedure called a sympathotomy, which interrupts the sympathetic signaling as opposed to destroying the ganglia.[39,41]

ETS has most commonly been used as an immediate and permanent treatment of primary palmar hyperhidrosis, although its use in the treatment of primary axillary hyperhidrosis shares those characteristics, with cure rates reportedly in the range of 96% for each location. Some patients have reported a decrease in plantar sweating following ETS even though this was not the intended target of the treatment.[10,30,31] This success has led some to suggest that early surgical treatment in children with severe primary palmar hyperhidrosis could avert the psychosocial and physical symptoms that are so disabling.[45]

Several studies support the use of ETS for severe palmar hyperhidrosis in children. One report published in 1995 looked at a period of 14 months where 23 ETS operations were performed on children aged 9 to 17. Intraoperative time was 12 to 25 minutes and uneventful for all patients. Most patients (18 of 23) had no postoperative difficulties and were sent home on postoperative Day 1. One patient developed a pneumothorax, was treated appropriately, and returned home on postoperative Day 3. All patients were able to resume their daily school routine 3 to 5 days following the procedure. Complete postprocedure satisfaction was obtained in 90% of those treated in up to 13 months of follow-up. There were two subjects (9%) who complained of moderate compensatory hyperhidrosis. A larger retrospective study published 1 year later (1996) examined patients aged 5.5 to 18 that were treated with ETS from 1992 to 1995 for severe primary palmar hyperhidrosis. Immediate and permanent resolution of palmar hyperhidrosis was observed in 98% of patients. Postoperative complications occurred in only two patients who developed pneumothorax that required 24-hour intercostal drainage.[45]

Another retrospective study conducted in the United Kingdom analyzed data from a total of 44 children (median age, 12.8 years) who underwent video-assisted thorascopic sympathectomy (85 total procedures) for the treatment of palmar hyperhidrosis over a 21-year period. The procedures performed included bilateral T2-T3 sympathectomy in 87% (38 of 44), bilateral T2-T5 sympathectomy in 9% (4 of 44), and right-sided thoracoscopic (left-sided done open) in 1% (0.5 of 44). Video-assisted thorascopic sympathectomy was not possible in 3% (1.5 of 44) of cases. Postoperative hospital stay ranged from 1 to 5 days (median, 2) and follow-up time ranged from 0.2 to 4.7 years (median, 1.3 years). During the follow-up period, 21% (9 of 44) of those treated developed severe hyperhidrosis of other parts of body (eg, plantar, axillary, or whole body). Postoperative complications were seen in about one-half (21 of 44) of those treated, which included postoperative pain (requiring >2 days hospital stay) in 18% (8 of 44), Horner syndrome in 18% (8 of 44), and recalcitrant palmar hyperhidrosis in 11% (5 of 44) of cases. Some patients (5 of 44) chose to repeat the procedure. Overall, the success rate for thoracoscopic sympathetectomy was 93% (79 of 85).[46]

Based on these and many other studies, video-assisted thorascopic sympathectomy seems to be an immediate and permanent treatment of severe palmar hyperhidrosis in children and adolescents that carries a low rate of morbidity and minimal risk for mortality. Some studies, however, do not have long-term follow-up regarding satisfaction with the outcome of the surgery or the degree and impact of compensatory hyperhidrosis on the patient. The compensatory hyperhidrosis has been characterized, at times, as a worse entity than the original hyperhidrosis for the patient.

CALCIUM-CHANNEL BLOCKERS, CLONIDINE, α-ADRENOCEPTOR ANTAGONISTS, BENZODIAZEPINE

Other medical treatments for hyperhidrosis have been tried with some success. Calcium-channel blockers, clonidine, and α-adrenoceptor antagonists have all been found to have efficacy in hyperhidrosis; however, these data are largely limited to isolated case reports and further research is needed to determine the appropriate role they should play in treating hyperhidrosis in children.[28] Another medical treatment involves benzodiazepine use for those patients whose hyperhidrosis is emotionally induced or anxiety driven. Physicians should be cautious when prescribing benzodiazepines in the pediatric population, however, because they can cause common side effects, such as dizziness, impaired coordination, and sedation, followed by dependency over the long term.[16,25]

SUMMARY

Primary hyperhidrosis often affects the psychological and social development of children, impacting quality of life, and can lead to profound emotional and social distress. Quality of life can be significantly improved by early diagnosis and therapy; however, underdiagnosis and lack of knowledge regarding therapeutic options has traditionally hindered maximization of therapy in the pediatric population. The current therapeutic options for primary pediatric hyperhidrosis, including topical and systemic therapies, iontophoresis, botulinum toxin injection, and surgical interventions, comprise an expanding knowledge regarding the management of hyperhidrosis in children and adolescents. Even though many different therapeutic options are available, further studies in the pediatric population are needed to help guide appropriate management.

REFERENCES

1. Fealey RD, Hebert AA. Disorders of the eccrine sweat glands and sweating. In: Goldsmith LA, Katz SI, Gilchrest BA, et al, editors. Fitzpatrick's dermatology in general medicine. 8th edition. New York: McGraw Hill; 2012. p. 936–47. Chapter 84.
2. Strutton DR, Kowalski JW, Glaser DA, et al. US prevalence of hyperhidrosis and impact on individuals with axillary hyperhidrosis: results from a national survey. J Am Acad Dermatol 2004;51:241–8.
3. Hamm H, Naumann MK, Kowalski JW, et al. Primary focal hyperhidrosis: disease characteristics and functional impairment. Dermatology 2006;212: 343–53.
4. Lear W, Kessler E, Solish N, et al. An epidemiological study of hyperhidrosis. Dermatol Surg 2007;33: S69–75.
5. Paller A, Shah P, Silverio A, et al. Oral glycopyrrolate as second-line treatment for primary pediatric hyperhidrosis. J Am Acad Dermatol 2012;67(5): 918–23.
6. Coutinho dos Santos LH, Gomes AM, Giraldi S, et al. Palmar hyperhidrosis: long-term follow-up of nine children and adolescents treated with botulinum toxin type A. Pediatr Dermatol 2009;26:439–44.
7. Gelbard CM, Epstein H, Hebert A. Primary pediatric hyperhidrosis: a review of current treatment options. Pediatr Dermatol 2008;25:591–8.
8. Walling HW. Primary hyperhidrosis increases the risk of cutaneous infection: a case-control study of 387 patients. J Am Acad Dermatol 2009;61:242–6.
9. Bellet JS. Diagnosis and treatment of primary focal hyperhidrosis in children and adolescents. Semin Cutan Med Surg 2010;29:121–6.
10. Cohen JL, Cohen G, Solish N. Diagnosis, impact, and management of focal hyperhidrosis: treatment review including botulinum toxin therapy. Facial Plast Surg Clin North Am 2007;15:17–30, v–vi.
11. Kreyden O, Böni R, Burg G. Hyperhidrosis and botulinum toxin in dermatology. Basel (Switzerland): Karger; 2001.
12. Shelley WB, Hurley HJ Jr. Studies on topical antiperspirant control of axillary hyperhidrosis. Acta Derm Venereol 1975;55:241–60.
13. Scholes KT, Crow KD, Ellis JP, et al. Axillary hyperhidrosis treated with alcoholic solution of aluminium chloride hexahydrate. Br Med J 1978;2:84–5.

14. Goh CL. Aluminum chloride hexahydrate versus palmar hyperhidrosis. Evaporimeter assessment. Int J Dermatol 1990;29:368–70.

15. Benohanian A, Dansereau A, Bolduc C, et al. Localized hyperhidrosis treated with aluminum chloride in a salicylic acid gel base. Int J Dermatol 1998;37:701–3.

16. Connolly M, de Berker D. Management of primary hyperhidrosis: a summary of the different treatment modalities. Am J Clin Dermatol 2003;4:681–97.

17. Stern LM. Preliminary study of glycopyrrolate in the management of drooling. J Paediatr Child Health 1997;33:52–4.

18. Blasco PA, Stansbury JC. Glycopyrrolate treatment of chronic drooling. Arch Pediatr Adolesc Med 1996;150:932–5.

19. Mijnhout GS, Kloosterman H, Simsek S, et al. Oxybutynin: dry days for patients with hyperhidrosis. Neth J Med 2006;64:326–8.

20. Matsui M, Yamada S, Oki T, et al. Functional analysis of muscarinic acetylcholine receptors using knockout mice. Life Sci 2004;75:2971–81.

21. Bajaj V, Langtry JA. Use of oral glycopyrronium bromide in hyperhidrosis. Br J Dermatol 2007;157:118–21.

22. Seukeran DC, Highet AS. The use of topical glycopyrrolate in the treatment of hyperhidrosis. Clin Exp Dermatol 1998;23:204–5.

23. Luh JY, Blackwell TA. Craniofacial hyperhidrosis successfully treated with topical glycopyrrolate. South Med J 2002;95:756–8.

24. Shaw JE, Abbott CA, Tindle K, et al. A randomised controlled trial of topical glycopyrrolate, the first specific treatment for diabetic gustatory sweating. Diabetologia 1997;40:299–301.

25. Haider A, Solish N. Focal hyperhidrosis: diagnosis and management. CMAJ 2005;172:69–75.

26. Kumar M, Foreman R, Berk D, et al. Oral glycopyrrolate for refractory pediatric and adolescent hyperhidrosis. Pediatr Dermatol 2014;31:e28–30.

27. Diaz L, Bicknel L, McNiece K, et al. Poster presentation. Society for Pediatric Dermatology Poster Presentation. Milwaukee (WI), July 11-14, 2013.

28. Eisenach JH, Atkinson JL, Fealey RD. Hyperhidrosis: evolving therapies for a well-established phenomenon. Mayo Clin Proc 2005;80:657–66.

29. Dolianitis C, Scarff CE, Kelly J, et al. Iontophoresis with glycopyrrolate for the treatment of palmoplantar hyperhidrosis. Australas J Dermatol 2004;45:208–12.

30. Karakoc Y, Aydemir EH, Kalkan MT, et al. Safe control of palmoplantar hyperhidrosis with direct electrical current. Int J Dermatol 2002;41:602–5.

31. Jeganathan R, Jordan S, Jones M, et al. Bilateral thoracoscopic sympathectomy: results and long-term follow-up. Interact Cardiovasc Thorac Surg 2008;7:67–70.

32. Baumann LS, Halem ML. Botulinum toxin-B and the management of hyperhidrosis. Clin Dermatol 2004;22:60–5.

33. Reisfeld R, Berliner KI. Evidence-based review of the nonsurgical management of hyperhidrosis. Thorac Surg Clin 2008;18:157–66.

34. Vazquez-Lopez ME, Pego-Reigosa R. Palmar hyperhidrosis in a 13-year-old boy: treatment with botulinum toxin A. Clin Pediatr (Phila) 2005;44:549–51.

35. Lowe NJ, Glaser DA, Eadie N, et al. Botulinum toxin type A in the treatment of primary axillary hyperhidrosis: a 52-week multicenter double-blind, randomized, placebo-controlled study of efficacy and safety. J Am Acad Dermatol 2007;56:604–11.

36. Glaser DA, Coleman WP, Loss R, et al. 4-Year longitudinal data on the efficacy and safety of repeated botulinum toxin type A therapy for primary axillary hyperhidrosis. Presented at the 65th American Academy of Dermatology Conference 2007. Washington, DC, February 1–5, 2007.

37. Bhakta BB, Roussounnis SH. Treating childhood hyperhidrosis with botulinum toxin type A. Arch Dis Child 2002;86:68.

38. Farrugia MK, Nicholls EA. Intradermal botulinum A toxin injection for axillary hyperhydrosis. J Pediatr Surg 2005;40:1668–9, 414.

39. Ram R, Lowe NJ, Yamauchi PS. Current and emerging therapeutic modalities for hyperhidrosis, part 2: moderately invasive and invasive procedures. Cutis 2007;79:281–8.

40. Commons G, Lim A. Treatment of axillary hyperhidrosis/bromidrosis using VASER ultrasound. Aesthetic Plast Surg 2009;33(3):312–23.

41. Moya J, Ramos R, Morera R, et al. Thoracic sympathicolysis for primary hyperhidrosis: a review of 918 procedures. Surg Endosc 2006;20:598–602.

42. Kestenholz PB, Weder W. Thoracic sympathectomy. Curr Probl Dermatol 2002;30:64–76.

43. Cohen Z, Shinar D, Levi I, et al. Thoracoscopic upper thoracic sympathectomy for primary palmar hyperhidrosis in children and adolescents. J Pediatr Surg 1995;30:471–3.

44. Steiner Z, Cohen Z, Kleiner O, et al. Do children tolerate thoracoscopic sympathectomy better than adults? Pediatr Surg Int 2007;24:343–7.

45. Cohen Z, Shinhar D, Mordechai J, et al. Thoracoscopic upper thoracic sympathectomy for primary palmar hyperhidrosis. Harefuah 1996;131:303–5.

46. Sinha C, Kiely E. Thoracoscopic sympathectomy for palmar hyperhidrosis in children: 21 years of experience at a tertiary care center. Eur J Pediatr Surg 2013;23:486–9.

Topical Therapies in Hyperhidrosis Care

David M. Pariser, MD[a,b,*], Angela Ballard, RN[a]

KEYWORDS

- Antiperspirants • Hyperhidrosis topical treatments • Topical glycopyrrolate • Aluminum chloride
- Aluminum salts • Aluminum chloride hexahydrate • Aluminum zirconium trichlorohydrex

KEY POINTS

- When used correctly, topical treatments for primary focal hyperhidrosis can provide significant benefit and, with patient education on usage, skin irritation can be limited and tolerable.
- Topical agents are a useful adjunct to other treatments such as onabotulinumtoxinA.
- Antiperspirants are most effective when applied to thoroughly dried skin at night.
- Many insurance companies consider treatment of hyperhidrosis with iontophoresis or onabotulinumtoxinA medically necessary only when topical aluminum chloride or other extrastrength antiperspirants are ineffective or result in a severe rash.
- Knowledge of the appropriate use of topical treatments is important for patient care on multiple levels.

PRIMARY HYPERHIDROSIS
The Nature of the Problem

Hyperhidrosis, also known as excessive sweating, is a dermatologic disorder characterized by sweating that is beyond what is anticipated or necessary for thermoregulation in the person's environment.[1] Primary, or idiopathic, hyperhidrosis and secondary hyperhidrosis are the chief categories of the condition.[2] Primary hyperhidrosis (hyperhidrosis that is not caused by another medical condition or as a side effect of medication) presents in approximately 3% of the population.[3] The excessive sweating experienced by people with primary hyperhidrosis is most often manifested at a focal body region such as on the palms, on the soles of the feet, in the axillae, or (less frequently) in the craniofacial region.[3] Patients with primary hyperhidrosis often experience focal excessive sweating at more than one of the body locations listed earlier.

Hyperhidrosis is of great concern to patients because of its physical, occupational, psychological, and social impacts on quality of life. For instance, patients with hyperhidrosis report physical discomfort caused by wet clothing and shoes.[1] In addition, skin maceration from persistent wetness can lead to bacterial and fungal overgrowth. This overgrowth can then cause intertrigo in the axillae as well as bromhidrosis (foul-smelling sweat), pitted keratolysis (an infection of the plantar surface characterized by pits or craters), and gram-negative bacterial infection and macerative infection of the feet.[4] From a practical and economic standpoint, excessive sweat can stain and eventually destroy clothing and shoes.[5] Patients may need to spend thousands of dollars annually for dry-cleaning and clothing replacement.[6]

Disclosure: Dr D.M. Pariser has been an investigator for Allergan, Dermira, and Watson Laboratories. Ms A. Ballard has no disclosures.
[a] International Hyperhidrosis Society, Quakertown, PA 18951, USA; [b] Department of Dermatology, Eastern Virginia Medical School, 601 Medical Tower, Norfolk, VA 23507, USA
* Corresponding author. Department of Dermatology, Eastern Virginia Medical School, 601 Medical Tower, Norfolk, VA 23507.
E-mail address: dpariser@pariserderm.com

Dermatol Clin 32 (2014) 485–490
http://dx.doi.org/10.1016/j.det.2014.06.008
0733-8635/14/$ – see front matter © 2014 Elsevier Inc. All rights reserved.

derm.theclinics.com

Psychosocial ramifications can be severe because of patient's embarrassment and the cultural stigma associated with sweating. Stereotypes regarding the causes of sweating (other than as a reaction to heat or exercise) may include nervousness, incompetence at a task, lack of cleanliness, or dishonesty. Day-to-day lives are also affected severely by excessive sweating; patients may find that their activities of daily living are negatively affected such that simple tasks become difficult, and household, educational, or job-related tools and documents may become damaged by wetness. Baseline evaluation of a series of patients treated for axillary hyperhidrosis found that 90% of the group reported an effect on their emotional status, and more than 70% had to change clothes 2 or more times per day.[7] More than 50% of patients with axillary hyperhidrosis identified in a US national consumer survey reported feeling less confident, 38% said they became frustrated by some daily activities, 34% were unhappy, and 20% said they were depressed.[8]

Palmar hyperhidrosis can interfere with activities of daily living as well as with occupational tasks. Having sweaty palms makes it difficult to grip tools, play musical instruments, and use electronic devices, and paper can be stained and ink smeared by dripping sweat.[1,5] Patients experiencing palmar excessive sweating have reported difficulty writing or drawing, frequent electric shocks, and dropping glass objects.[9] Occupational problems for those with axillary or generalized hyperhidrosis include needing to change clothes frequently and anxiety regarding presentations in front of audiences because of sweat-stained clothing and resultant embarrassment.[10] In the US national consumer survey mentioned earlier, 13% of patients with axillary hyperhidrosis reported a related decrease in work time.[8]

PATIENT EVALUATION OVERVIEW

The first step when evaluating a patient presenting with hyperhidrosis is a detailed clinical history with a focus on features of primary hyperhidrosis in order to support the diagnosis of primary focal hyperhidrosis (**Box 1**). It is also critical to know the patient's medical and surgical history as well as any medications, supplements, or complementary therapies that have been used. Review of systems should focus on the endocrine and neurologic systems. Physical examination includes an inspection for signs of excess sweating and/or related skin breakdown but such symptoms may not reliably be present.[3] Laboratory testing is usually not required.[3] The Hyperhidrosis Disease Severity Scale (HDSS) is a quick diagnostic tool providing

---

Box 1
Diagnostic features of primary hyperhidrosis

- Excessive sweating occurring in at least 1 of the following sites: axillae, palms, soles, or craniofacial region
- At least 6 months' duration
- Without apparent secondary causes (eg, medications, endocrine disease, neurologic disease)
- Including 2 or more of the following characteristics:

  Bilateral and approximately symmetric

  Age of onset less than 25 years

  Frequency of episodes at least once per week

  Positive family history

  Cessation of excessive sweating on sleep

  Impairment of daily activities

Adapted from Hornberger J, Grimes K, Naumann M, et al. Recognition, diagnosis, and treatment of primary focal hyperhidrosis. J Am Acad Dermatol 2004; 51(2):274–86

---

insight into the impact of hyperhidrosis on the patient's life (**Box 2**). The results can be used to tailor treatment and for insurance reimbursement or coverage documentation purposes.[3]

TOPICAL OPTIONS FOR HYPERHIDROSIS TREATMENT

Because of the history of safety, cost-effectiveness, and ease of use and access of topical therapies, and because many patients

---

Box 2
HDSS

How would you rate the severity of your hyperhidrosis?

1. My sweating is never noticeable and never interferes with my daily activities
2. My sweating is tolerable but sometimes interferes with my daily activities
3. My sweating is barely tolerable and frequently interferes with my daily activities
4. My sweating is intolerable and always interferes with my daily activities

From Walling HW, Swick BL. Treatment options for hyperhidrosis. Am J Clin Dermatol 2011;12:285–96; with permission.

obtain symptom relief from them, topical treatments are often the first line of treatment of primary focal hyperhidrosis (**Fig. 1**).[3] Topical antiperspirants are most effective for axillary sweating but may also be used for the palms of the hands, soles of the feet, and on the craniofacial area. Aluminum chloride is the most commonly used topical agent.[3]

ALUMINUM SALTS

Aluminum chloride is the partially neutralized form used in cosmetic antiperspirants, whereas aluminum chloride hexahydrate is used in prescription products and is among the most effective antiperspirants available.[11] Newer over-the-counter (OTC) clinical-strength antiperspirants are also available and are discussed later in this article.

With regard to mechanism of action, several studies have shown that aluminum salts cause an obstruction of the distal eccrine sweat gland ducts.[12] The mechanism underlying this obstruction is thought to be that the metal ions precipitate with mucopolysaccharides, damaging epithelial cells along the lumen of the duct and forming a plug that blocks sweat output (**Fig. 2**).[11] Sweat may still be produced, as shown by the appearance of miliaria (prickly heat) during heat stress, with sweat building up behind the obstruction created by the metallic salt.[12] However, normal sweat gland function returns with epidermal renewal, so retreatment/topical reapplication is required, with frequency depending on the product.[11] However, long-term histologic studies of eccrine glands in patients on chronic aluminum salt treatment have shown destruction of some secretory cells, accounting for the clinical finding of reduced severity of hyperhidrosis over time, as reflected by the need for less-frequent treatments.[12] Other metallic salts such as zirconium,

vanadium, and indium are thought to work by the same mechanism.[11] Some of these salts are more effective than aluminum salts, but aluminum salts have been used for more than 80 years and are inexpensive, easily available, and nontoxic, so they remain the common active ingredient of most preparations.[11]

Less severe cases of hyperhidrosis may respond to OTC aluminum chloride antiperspirants. More severe cases may require prescription-strength aluminum chloride (20% solution).[3] Most patients with hyperhidrosis note a reduction or cessation of sweating at night. In order for the plugs to form most efficiently, to limit skin irritation, increase efficacy, and limit damage to clothing, antiperspirants should be applied at nighttime, before bed, to dry skin. Clinical efficacy is often noted in 1 to 2 weeks.[3] However, compliance with nighttime application can be limited by the products having traditionally been part of the morning grooming routine. Fragrances may also interfere with sleep and patients may not think that the product is working during the day because there are no awareness signals that the product is still present in the morning.

In a study involving 691 patients with axillary hyperhidrosis treated with aluminum chloride, 82% of the group reported dryness or a tolerable amount of sweating, and, in longer follow-up, 87% reported satisfaction with the treatment.[11] In that study, various concentrations were evaluated, and the investigators concluded that a 15% solution was as effective as 20% solution and was better tolerated.[11]

Palmar hyperhidrosis is less responsive to aluminum chloride therapy than axillary hyperhidrosis[13] and successful treatment may require active ingredient concentrations up to 30%.[14]

Skin irritation is a common limiting factor in the treatment of hyperhidrosis with aluminum chloride. A study of 38 patients with axillary hyperhidrosis reported treatment-limiting irritation in 26% of patients.[15] The most common adverse effects of aluminum chloride treatment are itching and stinging immediately after application, and ongoing skin irritation.[11] In one series of 691 patients, pruritus was minor and short in duration in 70% of study participants, moderate in 21%, and severe in 9%, whereas skin irritation was moderate in 36% and severe in 14%. During maintenance treatment, less itching and skin irritation were seen.[11] In many cases, skin irritation is mild and can be controlled with the application of 1% hydrocortisone cream the morning after treatment.[16] Damage to fabrics can occur, so patients should be counseled against wearing expensive nightwear.[14]

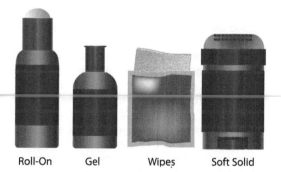

Roll-On   Gel   Wipes   Soft Solid

Fig. 1. Topical treatments are often the first line of treatment of primary focal hyperhidrosis. (*Courtesy of* Albert Ganss, International Hyperhidrosis Society, Quakertown, PA; with permission.)

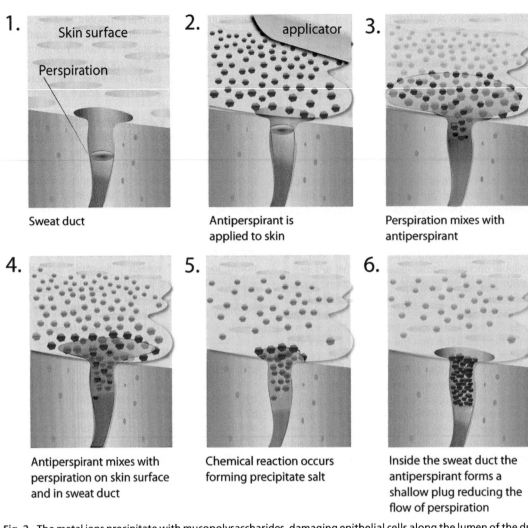

1. Skin surface

Perspiration

Sweat duct

2. applicator

Antiperspirant is applied to skin

3. Perspiration mixes with antiperspirant

4. Antiperspirant mixes with perspiration on skin surface and in sweat duct

5. Chemical reaction occurs forming precipitate salt

6. Inside the sweat duct the antiperspirant forms a shallow plug reducing the flow of perspiration

Fig. 2. The metal ions precipitate with mucopolysaccharides, damaging epithelial cells along the lumen of the duct and forming a plug that blocks sweat output. (*Courtesy of* Albert Ganss, International Hyperhidrosis Society, Quakertown, PA; with permission.)

Available by prescription, 20% aluminum hexahydrate in anhydrous ethanol (Drysol, Person and Covey, Inc, Glendale, CA) is a commonly used agent.[5] Concentrations of 10% to 15% and up to 30% are used in compounded formulations to treat axillary and palmoplantar hyperhidrosis, respectively.[14]

Following a recommended regimen may enhance efficacy and reduce the incidence of adverse effects.[13] Aluminum chloride should remain on the skin for 6 to 8 hours to be effective. Overnight application best takes advantage of low sweat output during sleep because diffusion of the aluminum ions into the sweat gland may be negatively affected if the gland is actively excreting sweat.[11] As mentioned earlier, patients need to be educated that, despite nighttime application, the product continues to work during the day and that adjustment of the morning grooming routine is necessary. Those patients who may want to use a fragranced product as part of morning grooming can be instructed to use a nonmedicated deodorant in the morning after a bath or shower.

If the patient regularly shaves the axillary region, it is best to wait 24 to 48 hours after shaving before applying the medication to decrease irritation.[13] Irritating hydrochloric acid forms in the presence of water, so prewashing is not advised; drying the axillae with a blow dryer may reduce irritation.[13] In the morning, the medication should be washed off before daytime sweating begins.[13] Irritated skin can be treated with topical hydrocortisone cream for up to 2 weeks if irritation persists.[5] If irritation persists beyond that point, a dermatology consult should be obtained. Nightly treatments are recommended until an effect is noted, and then the interval between treatments can be lengthened.[5]

In another study, 4% salicylic acid in a hydro-alcoholic gel base was used as the vehicle for aluminum chloride hexahydrate in 238 patients with hyperhidrosis involving the axillae, feet, hands, and groin.[17] The rationale for using this combination included possible enhancement of aluminum chloride absorption, possible additional antiperspirant effects of salicylic acid, and potentially less skin irritation afforded by the hydroalcoholic gel. The percentage of aluminum chloride varied with the site treated: 10% to 25% for the axillae and 30% to 40% for the palms and soles. For patients with axillary disease, 94% reported excellent to good results. Excellent to good results were reported by 60% and 84% of patients with palmar or plantar involvement, respectively. Patients who had previously failed to respond to aluminum chloride in absolute alcohol or who could not tolerate it seemed to improve with use of the salicylic acid gel vehicle. The researchers suggested further study on this treatment option.[16]

TOPICAL GLYCOPYRROLATE

Glycopyrrolate is an anticholinergic agent that is used off-label systemically for the treatment of hyperhidrosis. Topical glycopyrrolate may also be effective for focal hyperhidrosis. A topical application of 0.5% or 1% glycopyrrolate was studied in 16 patients with Frey syndrome (gustatory hyperhidrosis) and was effective and free of adverse effects.[18] In another study of 25 patients with craniofacial sweating, all the patients had half their foreheads treated with 2% glycopyrrolate and the other half treated with placebo. This split-face study found that 96% of the patients were satisfied with the effectiveness; whereas 1 patient did not tolerate the regimen because of headache. Improvement was transient, lasting 1 to 2 days for most patients.[19] Topical glycopyrrolate may also be considered as a treatment option for large areas of sweating (ie, post-ETS compensatory sweating) with side effects being mydriasis and accommodation failure,[20] and urinary retention.[21] In another uncontrolled study in which 35 patients with axillary hyperhidrosis who previously failed treatment with topical aluminum chloride applied a topical formulation of 1% glycopyrrolate in ceto-macrogol cream BP once daily for 1 month found less favorable results.[22] Only 9 patients had a greater than 50% reduction in the Dermatology Life Quality Index score, and only 2 patients desired to continue treatment at the end of the study. The investigators of the study commented that their clinical experience with this formulation of topical glycopyrrolate was more favorable in patients with craniofacial hyperhidrosis.

Topical glycopyrrolate is not commercially available worldwide, but can be compounded. A commercial product is not available in the United States.

Topical agents such as glutaraldehyde, formaldehyde, and tannic acid are currently seldom used because of irritancy, skin discoloration, and the availability of alternatives.[3]

CLINICAL-STRENGTH OTC PRODUCTS

A new generation of OTC antiperspirants includes aluminum zirconium trichlorohydrex and may be an option for nonaxillary as well as axillary hyperhidrosis. These products provide more sweat-reduction benefits than traditional OTC products with less reported irritation to the skin than prescription topical therapies.[23] In a study of 20 male participants published in 2012, researchers found that sweat reduction caused by the use of an OTC clinical-strength antiperspirant product was more effective (an average of 34% better) than typical prescription topical (6.5%) aluminum chloride treatments with less skin irritation. OTC clinical-strength antiperspirants are typically based on partially neutralized salts such as aluminum zirconium trichlorohydrate gly. These materials reduce the amount of HCl (which is blamed for skin irritation) produced on the skin by as much as 80%, create a more superficial duct blockage than aluminum chloride, and allow daily or twice-daily application without significant skin irritation (which patients tend to find appealing and which fits into patients' traditional grooming routines). Although blockages are more superficial than may occur with stronger aluminum chloride solutions, there are several literature reports indicating that the blockage lasts more than 7 days, so it is possible to achieve high sweat-reduction values provided the active agent is effectively delivered to the opening of the eccrine gland daily.[24] Thus OTC clinical-strength soft-solid antiperspirants may be considered as an alternative treatment to aluminum chloride antiperspirants for the treatment of excessive sweating.

Because of information on the Internet, some patients ask about the association of aluminum use and Alzheimer disease and breast cancer. The Alzheimer's Association, the American Cancer Society, the Susan B. Komen Cancer Foundation, and the National Cancer Institute have statements on their respective Web sites indicating that there is no research to support claims that antiperspirant use is linked to either Alzheimer or breast cancer risk or incidence.

In conclusion, when used correctly, topical treatments for primary focal hyperhidrosis can provide significant benefit and, with patient education on usage, skin irritation can be limited and tolerable for some patients. Topical agents may also be a useful adjunct to other treatments such as onabotulinumtoxinA and systemic therapies. Many insurance companies consider treatment of hyperhidrosis with iontophoresis or onabotulinumtoxinA medically necessary only when topical aluminum chloride or other extrastrength antiperspirants are ineffective, result in a severe irritation, or produce other complications. Appropriate use of topical treatments is important for almost all patients with hyperhidrosis.

REFERENCES

1. Atkins JL, Butler PE. Hyperhidrosis: a review of current management. Plast Reconstr Surg 2002;110:222–8.
2. Böni R. Generalized hyperhidrosis and its systemic treatment. Curr Probl Dermatol 2002;30:44–7.
3. Walling HW, Swick BL. Treatment options for hyperhidrosis. Am J Clin Dermatol 2011;12:285–95.
4. Hölzle E. Pathophysiology of sweating. Curr Probl Dermatol 2002;30:10–22.
5. Stolman LP. Treatment of hyperhidrosis. Dermatol Clin 1998;16:863–9.
6. Glogau RG. Botulinum A neurotoxin for axillary hyperhidrosis. No sweat Botox. Dermatol Surg 1998;24:817–9.
7. Naumann MK, Hamm H, Lowe NJ. Effect of botulinum toxin type A on quality of life measures in patients with excessive axillary sweating: a randomized controlled trial. Br J Dermatol 2002;147:1218–26.
8. Strutton DR, Kowalski J, Glaser DA, et al. Impact of daily activities in the US for individuals with axillary hyperhidrosis: results from a national consumer panel. Poster presented at: 61st annual meeting of the American Academy of Dermatology. San Francisco (CA), March 21-26, 2003.
9. Adar R, Kurchin A, Zweig A, et al. Palmar hyperhidrosis and its surgical treatment: a report of 100 cases. Ann Surg 1977;186:34–41.
10. Davidson JR, Foa EB, Connor KM, et al. Hyperhidrosis in social anxiety disorder. Prog Neuropsychopharmacol Biol Psychiatry 2002;26:1327–31.
11. Hölzle E. Topical pharmacological treatment. Curr Probl Dermatol 2002;30:30–43.
12. Hölzle E, Braun-Falco O. Structural changes in axillary eccrine glands following long-term treatment with aluminum chloride hexahydrate solution. Br J Dermatol 1984;110:399–403.
13. White JW Jr. Treatment of primary hyperhidrosis. Mayo Clin Proc 1986;61:951–6.
14. Tögel B, Greve B, Raulin C. Current therapeutic strategies for hyperhidrosis: a review. Eur J Dermatol 2002;12:219–23.
15. Glent-Madsen L, Dahl JC. Axillary hyperhidrosis: local treatment with aluminum-chloride hexahydrate 25% in absolute ethanol with and without supplementary treatment with triethanolamine. Acta Derm Venereol 1988;68:87–9.
16. Scholes KT. Axillary hyperhidrosis. Br Med J 1978;2:773.
17. Benohanian A, Dansereau A, Bolduc C, et al. Localized hyperhidrosis treated with aluminum chloride in a salicylic acid gel base. Int J Dermatol 1998;37:701–3.
18. Hays LL. The Frey syndrome: a review and double blind evaluation of the topical use of a new anticholinergic agent. Laryngoscope 1978;88:1796–824.
19. Kim WO, Kil HK, Yoon KB, et al. Topical glycopyrrolate for patients with facial hyperhidrosis. Br J Dermatol 2008;158:1094–7.
20. Izadi S, Choudhary A, Newman W. Mydriasis and accommodative failure from exposure to topical glycopyrrolate used in hyperhidrosis. J Neuroophthalmol 2006;26:232–3.
21. Madan V, Beck MH. Urinary retention caused by topical glycopyrrolate for hyperhidrosis. Br J Dermatol 2006;155:634–5.
22. Mackenzie A, Burns C, Kavanagh G. Topical glycopyrrolate for axillary hyperhidrosis. Br J Dermatol 2013;169:483.
23. Thomas M, et al. "Alternative topical treatment to an aluminum chloride antiperspirant that provides prescription strength efficacy with significantly less irritation", presented at the 65th Annual Meeting of the American Academy of Dermatology. Washington, DC, February 2–6, 2007.
24. Swaile DF, Elstun LT, Benzing KW. Clinical studies of sweat rate reduction by an over-the-counter soft-solid antiperspirant and comparison with a prescription antiperspirant product in male panelists. Br J Dermatol 2012;166(Suppl 1):22–6.

Iontophoresis for Palmar and Plantar Hyperhidrosis

David M. Pariser, MD[a,b,*], Angela Ballard, RN[a]

KEYWORDS

- Hyperhidrosis • Hyperhidrosis treatments • Iontophoresis • Palmar hyperhidrosis
- Plantar hyperhidrosis • Palmoplantar hyperhidrosis • Excessive sweating

KEY POINTS

- Iontophoresis has a long history of safe and effective use.
- Once a home device is obtained and the patient has received adequate education and training, the maintenance cost and effort are minimal for the patient and health care provider, alike.
- Iontophoresis should not be overlooked as a primary treatment of palmar and plantar hyperhidrosis.

Iontophoresis has been used to treat palmar hyperhidrosis (**Fig. 1**) and plantar hyperhidrosis (**Fig. 2**) for more than 70 years. Although its mechanism of action is still not entirely understood, iontophoresis has proved to provide reliable, effective treatment when practiced with appropriate technique, timing, and tweaks (as necessary). Patients who prefer to manage their excessive sweating treatment at home may find that, after they have learned the treatment process from a health care professional, iontophoresis is a particularly attractive option. In addition, many health insurance programs consider treatment with iontophoresis for hyperhidrosis medically necessary when antiperspirants have been ineffective or have resulted in a skin irritation.

Iontophoresis is the passing of an ionized substance through intact skin by the application of a direct electrical current.[1] In most cases, simple tap water and an iontophoresis medical device are all that is required to achieve sweat relief, and many dermatologists consider the treatment to be first line to address primary focal palmar or plantar hyperhidrosis.[1,2] In some situations, adjustments to the regimen may be necessary (eg, adding baking soda or an anticholinergic to the water); these are discussed later. Three iontophoresis

devices are available in the United States, and registered with the US Food and Drug Administration for the treatment of hyperhidrosis. These devices are the R.A. Fischer (both MD-1a and MD-2 models) and the Drionic.

As mentioned earlier, studies have not yet fully explained the provenance of the efficacy of ontophoresis. However, there are several theories, including the plugging of sweat glands as a result of ion deposition,[3] a blocking of sympathetic nerve transmission,[2] or a decrease in pH as a result of accumulation of hydrogen ions.[4]

EFFICACY

Regardless of why it works, studies have shown that iontophoresis does provide relief from excessive sweating symptoms for many patients. For instance, an early (1952) observational study of iontophoresis in 113 patients with palmoplantar hyperhidrosis[5] reported a response rate of 91% and showed that adding ionizable agents to the water did not improve the results.

In a study published in 1987, 18 patients with palmar hyperhidrosis were treated with iontophoresis for 1 hand, and the other hand served as the control. These patients were treated with 12 to

[a] International Hyperhidrosis Society, Quakertown, PA 18951, USA; [b] Department of Dermatology, Eastern Virginia Medical School, 601 Medical Tower, Norfolk, VA 23507, USA
* Corresponding author. Department of Dermatology, Eastern Virginia Medical School, 601 Medical Tower, Norfolk, VA 23507.
E-mail address: dpariser@pariserderm.com

Dermatol Clin 32 (2014) 491–494
http://dx.doi.org/10.1016/j.det.2014.06.009
0733-8635/14/$ – see front matter © 2014 Elsevier Inc. All rights reserved.

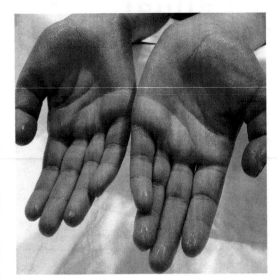

Fig. 1. Severe palmar hyperhidrosis for treatment by iontophoresis. (*Courtesy of* Albert Ganss, International Hyperhidrosis Society, Quakertown, PA; with permission.)

20 mA for 20 minutes, 3 times a week, for 3 weeks. The results showed that 15 of 18 participants had markedly reduced sweat production in their treated hands.[6]

In addition, a 1989 controlled trial with 11 patients randomized to actual or sham procedures reported 81% reduction in sweat production measured by gravimeter after a median of 10 treatments. The symptom improvement was thereafter maintained with treatment every other week.[7] Similarly, a 2002 controlled trial of 112 patients diagnosed with palmar hyperhidrosis showed that, after 8 treatments, sweating was reduced 81.2% from baseline. This reduction was seen 20 days after the eighth treatment, with the mean return of symptoms occurring at 35 days.[8]

ADVERSE EVENTS

Adverse events from iontophoresis are usually mild and do not necessitate termination of the treatment. Often, proper technique and education of the patient can prevent adverse events and side effects. For instance, to prevent mild shocks, patients should be reminded to keep their hands or feet in the water trays while the device is in use and to avoid touching the electrodes.[1] Scratches and cuts on the surface of the area to be treated should be covered with a thin layer of petroleum jelly.[1,9] Petroleum jelly may also be applied along the water line to help prevent erythema of that region.

Vesiculation in the affected area has been reported, but is usually transient.[6] Eight of 112 patients reported vesiculation in a 2002 study.[8]

Redness of the skin, often along the water line, is also commonly reported.[6] Twelve of 122 patients reported erythema in the 2002 study.[8]

Both erythema and vesiculation can be treated with 1% hydrocortisone cream, if these symptoms persist. Prevention may be achieved via petroleum jelly application.[1]

Discomfort, either as a burning sensation or pins and needles, is also common. All patients in 1 series complained of pins and needles, and 20 of 112 complained of the burning sensation.[6,8]

Sometimes, the treatment area may become dry, cracked, or fissured. In these instances, moisturizers or decreasing the frequency of iontophoresis sessions may be necessary.[1]

CONTRAINDICATIONS

Women who are pregnant or people with pacemakers or substantial metal implants (in the path of the electrical current, such as joint replacements), cardiac conditions, or epilepsy should not use iontophoresis.

RECOMMENDED REGIMEN

Iontophoresis treatment usually begins in the clinic under the direction and care of a health care professional. Once the desired results have been achieved, or it seems that the patient has a clear understanding of iontophoresis and has gained the necessary know-how, the health care provider may determine that they are ready to perform treatments at home using a device purchased or rented for that purpose.

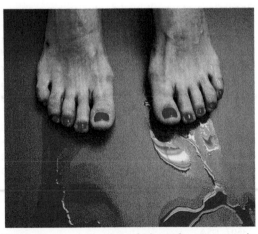

Fig. 2. Severe plantar hyperhidrosis for treatment by iontophoresis. (*Courtesy of* Albert Ganss, International Hyperhidrosis Society, Quakertown, PA; and Adelaide Hebert, MD, University of Texas, Houston, TX; with permission.)

As mentioned earlier, apply petroleum jelly with a cotton swab to cover any cuts on hands or feet before immersing them in the water trays/baths. To relieve skin irritation that may have already occurred, apply 1% hydrocortisone cream after treatment.

Initially, iontophoresis treatments are required on a more frequent basis. It is often recommended that treatments begin with a Monday, Wednesday, and Friday schedule until the condition improves. Then, the treatments can be tapered down to once per week. Once per week seems to be ideal in terms of maintaining effectiveness and limiting inconvenience to the patient.

Use regular tap water.[2] Fill the trays with just enough water to cover the hands (**Fig. 3**A) or feet (see **Fig. 3**B) or 1 hand and 1 foot (see **Fig. 3**C).[1]

After placing the body part in the device tray, turn the machine on. Slowly increase the amperage until a tingling that is not unpleasant is felt in the affected area,[9] or to a maximum of 20 mA.[1] To start, treat for 20 minutes a session every 2 to 3 days.[1] Halfway through the 20-minute session, reverse current flow to switch anode site to opposite side.[1] Frequency of maintenance treatment varies, but 1 to 3 times a week is usually necessary.[2]

If mineral content of tap water is low (water may be termed as being too soft), insufficient current flow may occur. This situation can be corrected by adding 5 g (1 teaspoon) of baking soda to each tray.[1]

If a patient fails to respond to tap water iontophoresis alone, and after mineral content of the tap water has been addressed, consider adding an anticholinergic to the water trays, such as 2-mg tablets of glycopyrrolate (crushed). Adjust the dose based on efficacy or side effects.[1] In a study of 20 patients with palmar and plantar hyperhidrosis,[10] when glycopyrrolate was added to the iontophoresis water trays (bilateral/both trays, unilateral/1 side only, or tap water alone), dryness was achieved for 11 days (bilateral glycopyrrolate), 5 days (unilateral glycopyrrolate), and 3 days (tap water alone). It has been suggested that the bilateral glycopyrrolate was more effective because of greater systemic absorption of the anticholinergic.

Patients who do not respond to iontophoresis may be candidates for a combination therapy, such as an iontophoresis regimen combined with clinical strength over-the-counter antiperspirants or prescription antiperspirants applied at night, before bedtime (see article on related topical treatments for hyperhidrosis elsewhere in this issue by

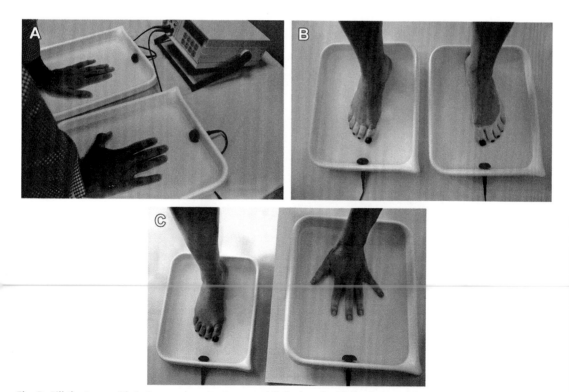

Fig. 3. Fill the trays with just enough water to cover (*A*) the hands, (*B*) the feet, or (*C*) 1 hand and 1 foot. (*Courtesy of* Albert Ganss, International Hyperhidrosis Society, Quakertown, PA; with permission.)

Pariser and Ballard). This mixed therapy can allow for less frequent iontophoresis treatment of patient convenience and compliance.

Iontophoresis has a long history of safe and effective use and, once a home device is obtained and the patient has received adequate education and training, the maintenance cost and effort are minimal for the patient and health care provider, alike. Thus, iontophoresis should not be overlooked as a primary treatment of palmar and plantar hyperhidrosis.

REFERENCES

1. Stolman LP. Treatment of hyperhidrosis. Dermatol Clin 1998;16:863–9.
2. Anliker MD, Kreyden OP. Tap water iontophoresis. Curr Probl Dermatol 2002;30:48–56.
3. Hill AC, Baker GF, Jansen GT. Mechanism of action of iontophoresis in the treatment of palmar hyperhidrosis. Cutis 1981;28:69–70, 72.
4. Wang L, Hilliges M, Gajecki M, et al. No change in skin innervations in patients with palmar hyperhidrosis treated with tap-water iontophoresis. Br J Dermatol 1994;131:742–3.
5. Bouman HD, Lentzer EM. The treatment of hyperhidrosis of hands and feet with constant current. Am J Phys Med 1952;31:158–69.
6. Stolman LP. Treatment of excess sweating of the palms by iontophoresis. Arch Dermatol 1987;123: 893–6.
7. Dahl JC, Glent-Madsen L. Treatment of hyperhidrosis manuum by tap water iontophoresis. Acta Derm Venereol 1989;69:346–8.
8. Karakoç Y, Aydemir EH, Kalkan MT, et al. Safe control of palmoplantar hyperhidrosis with direct electrical current. Int J Dermatol 2002;41:602–5.
9. Levit F. Treatment of hyperhidrosis by tap water iontophoresis. Cutis 1980;26:192–4.
10. Dolianitis C, Scarff CE, Kelly J, et al. Iontophoresis with glycopyrrolate for the treatment of palmoplantar hyperhidrosis. Australas J Dermatol 2004;45:208–12.

Botulinum Toxin for Axillary Hyperhidrosis

Ada Regina Trindade de Almeida, MD[a],*, Suelen Montagner, MD[b]

KEYWORDS

- Axillary hyperhidrosis • Excessive underarm sweating • Botox • Botulinum toxin • Neuromodulators

KEY POINTS

- Botulinum toxin has been proved to be safe and effective for the treatment of axillary hyperhidrosis.
- Although its pathophysiology continues to be controversial, the beneficial effect of type-A neuromodulators in temporarily inhibiting localized sweating supports a level A recommendation from evidence-based review.
- Before the procedure, the correct identification of the affected area is mandatory to avoid wastage of drug and neglect of target areas, and to enhance efficacy, as the hyperhidrotic location may not match the hairy axillary region.

INTRODUCTION

Axillary hyperhidrosis is a disease that affects the social and occupational lives of many people on all continents.[1,2] Axillary hyperhidrosis begins during the teenage years and equally affects men and women.[3] When associated with axillary malodor it is known as bromhidrosis.

The pathophysiology of primary focal hyperhidrosis is not well understood. It can result from hyperstimulation of eccrine and, possibly, apoeccrine sweat glands.[4]

Eccrine glands are distributed over almost the entire body surface[5] and are most numerous on the palms, soles, forehead, axillae, and cheeks.[6] Innervated by cholinergic postganglionic sympathetic nerve fibers, they excrete sweat and contribute to regulation of body temperature.[6,7] When comparing patients with excessive sweating with normal controls, histologic studies have not shown any morphologic alterations or increase in the number or size of the sweat glands.[8] However, preliminary findings of a recent study suggest that the eccrine gland's secretory clear cell exercises a main role in fluid transport (the only one equipped with cotransporter and aquaporin channels), and is likely the source of excessive sweating in this form of hyperhidrosis.[9]

Apocrine glands are stimulated by epinephrine and norepinephrine, and are specifically localized at the urogenital regions and the axillae.[9,10] These glands produce a viscid secretion that can become malodorous as a result of bacterial breakdown.[11]

Sato and colleagues[5,12] described apoeccrine glands in 1989 as having morphologic characteristics of both eccrine and apocrine types. According to these investigators, they correspond to 10% to 45% of all axillary glands and respond to cholinergic stimuli, and intensely so to epinephrine and isoproterenol infusion.[7] However, recent histologic studies have failed to show evidence of

Funding Sources: None.
Conflict of Interest: Dr A.R. Trindade de Almeida has been a consultant to Allergan, Inc and has participated in clinical trials for Allergan and Galderma; Dr S. Montagner has no conflicts of interest.
a Department of Dermatology, Hospital do Servidor Público Municipal de São Paulo (SP), Rua Turiaçu, 390, cjs 113-114, Perdizes, São Paulo, São Paulo 05005-000, Brazil; b Av. Eng. Carlos Stevenson, 885, Campinas, São Paulo 13092-132, Brazil
* Corresponding author.
E-mail address: artrindal@uol.com.br

derm.theclinics.com

apoeccrine glands in the tissues of the axillary region investigated.[8,9] The existence of these glands remains controversial.[9,13,14]

BOTULINUM TOXIN

Intracutaneous injections of botulinum toxin (BoNT) have been used as a treatment for focal hyperhidrosis since 1996 with safety, efficacy, and high levels of patient satisfaction.[2,15] Two types of botulinum toxins, BoNT type A (BoNT-A) and BoNT type B (BoNT-B), were studied in axillary hyperhidrosis, and both demonstrated effectiveness in temporarily inhibiting sweating, although acting at different target sites. BoNT-A binds to and cleaves the 25-kDa synaptosomal-associated protein (SNAP-25), whereas BoNT-B acts on the vesicle-associated membrane protein (VAMP or Synaptobrevin),[16,17] both blocking the release of acetylcholine from cholinergic neurons that innervate sweat glands.[16,18]

The use of BoNT-A for the treatment of axillary hyperhidrosis was approved in 2004 by the US Food and Drug Administration (FDA),[19] since then a multitude of studies have confirmed its efficacy, beneficial effects, and paucity of side effects.[20–24]

There are many commercial available BoNT-A products available worldwide. The formulations are not identical and present individual potencies, making caution necessary to ensure proper use. In April 2009, the FDA established drug names to reinforce these differences,[25] summarized in **Table 1**.

There is no globally accepted exact ratio among the different formulations. Reviewing the related published literature, the most commonly accepted dose correlation among products are: 1 U onabotulinumtoxinA (OnaA) = 1 U incobotulinumtoxinA (IncoA) = 1 U BoNT-A (Lanzou) = 1 U BoNT-A (Medytox) = 2,5–3 U abobotulinumtoxinA (AboA).

The available BoNT-B (rimabotulinumtoxinB [RimaB]) products are Neurobloc in the European Union and Myobloc in the United States. Unlike BoNT-A, it is not commercially available worldwide, and probably for this reason a limited number of studies of axillary hyperhidrosis being treated with this toxin type have been published. The literature found describes side effects related to distant spread of the toxin, such as dry eyes and dry mouth, which are not commonly described after the use of BoNT-A.[26–28] The dose correlation between BoNT-A and BoNT-B varies from 20 to 100 U of RimaB to 1 U of OnaA.[26–29]

A recent evidence-based review[30] of hypersecretory disorders that searched for botulinum toxin as a treatment of axillary hyperhidrosis found 2 Class I (prospective, randomized, controlled, and with masked outcome assessment clinical trial with strict requirements) studies (1 with OnaA[21] and 1 with AboA[20]) and 5 Class II (similar to Class I trials but lacking 1 or more of the required criteria) studies. The investigators concluded that the evidence supports a level A recommendation for BoNT-A in general and a level B recommendation for OnaA and AboA individually, whereas RimaB and IncoA received a level U recommendation (insufficient data) for axillary hyperhidrosis.

Some studies have compared the use of different toxins for the treatment of axillary hyperhidrosis.

Studies Comparing BoNT-A Products

Kalner[15] performed a prospective same-patient comparison between OnaA in one axilla and AboA in the other, using a conversion factor of 1 U OnaA to 3 U AboA. She noted that OnaA resulted in a faster onset of action, within 1 week,

Table 1		
Commercially available botulinum toxin A (BoNT-A)		
Botulinum Toxin	Trade Name	Origin
OnabotulinumtoxinA (OnaA)	Botox	(Allergan, Irvine, CA, USA)
AbobotulinumtoxinA (AboA)	Dysport	(Ipsen Biopharm, UK) in USA, Europe, and Latin America
BoNT-A	Prosigne	(Lanzhou, China) in Asia and Latin America
BoNT-A	Neuronox	(Medytox, South Korea) in Asia, Botulift in Latin America
IncobotulinumtoxinA (IncoA)	Xeomin	(Merz Pharma, Germany) in Canada, Germany, USA, Latin America
BoNT-A	PureTox	(Mentor Corp, Santa Barbara, CA, USA) uncomplexed BoNT-A. Phase III studies

versus 2 weeks for AboA. She also observed a longer duration of benefit (9 months), whereas the axilla treated with AboA maintained the results for 6 months.[15] In another comparative study performed in 2007 on 10 patients, Talarico-Filho and colleagues[31] did not find statistically significant differences in the onset of sweating reduction or the duration of benefit using the same conversion factor.

In a double-blind comparative study of 46 patients, Dressler[32] injected 50 U OnaA in one axilla and 50 U IncoA in the contralateral axilla. Both 100-U/vial products were reconstituted in 10 mL of saline (10 U/mL). He found no difference in efficacy, onset of action, duration, or side effects between the 2 formulations.

Studies Comparing BoNT-A and BoNT-B Products

In 2011, Frasson and colleagues[29] treated 10 patients using 2500 U of RimaB in one axilla and 50 U of OnaA in the contralateral axilla (50 U B:1 U A). BoNT-B was more effective than BoNT-A in reducing sweating production in the affected area, with faster onset, longer duration of benefit, and higher treatment satisfaction scores. No systemic adverse effects were described. According to the investigators, their findings differed from those found in the literature because other studies used lower toxin ratios (40:1 or 20:1) and higher dilutions.

Further studies are needed to standardize the treatment while aiming at reducing side effects and improving the benefits. The toxin type will be selected at the physician's discretion and according to its safety and product availability.

TOXIN SOLUTION

A recent review about botulinum toxin handling found that "there is no standardized dilution for BoNT-A treatment of focal hyperhidrosis."[16] Reported dilutions found in the literature vary from 1 to 10 mL of saline for OnaA (with most physicians using between 2 and 5 mL), whereas for AboA the reconstitution volumes vary from 1.25 to 10 mL (with the use of 2.5–5 mL being the most frequent). In the only study of IncoA for hyperhidrosis, the dilution used was 10 U/mL.[16] **Table 2** summarizes the dilution volumes described in the literature.

The authors prefer to reconstitute the 100-U vial of OnaA (Botox) in 2 mL saline, achieving a dose of 50 U/mL.

The same article previously quoted also mentions that different substances can be added to the toxin solution with no harm to the toxin, such as hyaluronidase, lidocaine, and epinephrine.

Table 2
Reported dilutions for hyperhidrosis

Toxin	Dilution Range (mL saline)	Most Commonly Used Dilution (mL)
OnabotulinumtoxinA	1–10	2–5
AbobotulinumtoxinA	1.25–10	2.5–5
IncobotulinumtoxinA	1–10	10 (1 paper)

Among these substances, the most interesting for axillary treatment is lidocaine. A recent double-blind, randomized, comparative study treated 8 patients with 50 U OnaA diluted in 0.5 mL saline plus 1 mL of 2% lidocaine into one axilla, and 50 U OnaA diluted in 1.5 mL saline into the other axilla.[33] Vadoud-Seyedi and Simonart[34] also treated 29 patients in a similar manner in 2007, with a dilution of 5 mL. Both studies showed equal effectiveness of BoNT-A reconstituted in saline or lidocaine. However, the toxin diluted in lidocaine caused less pain, and may be preferable for treating axillary hyperhidrosis.[33,34]

When reconstituted with saline admixed with hyaluronidase, OnaA has its efficacy maintained after 2 weeks and shows enhanced diffusion, as observed by Goodman[35] in 2003.

EVALUATION METHODS

After the selection of the toxin, it is important to identify the area to be treated. The Minor iodine-starch test is a useful method to map the extension of the affected area[36] in addition to the posttreatment residual sweating, but it does not provide accurate information on the amount of sweat produced.

The test is usually applied before any topical or regional anesthesia, and is cheap and easy to perform.[37] The first step is to dry the affected area with an absorbent paper. Then a 3% to 5% iodine solution is applied to the underarm and neighboring region and is allowed to dry. In some patients, the continuous sweat must be wiped again just before the starch application to avoid false reactions (**Fig. 1**). In contact with starch plus iodine, the sweat acquires a dark purple color, being clearly visible. One must be aware that the commercial povidone-iodine topical solution with 10% iodopovidone contains only 1% free iodine. Therefore, when using this agent the Minor test results might not be satisfactory.[38]

Another important detail to observe is that the axillary hyperhidrotic area very often does not coincide with the hairy underarm region.

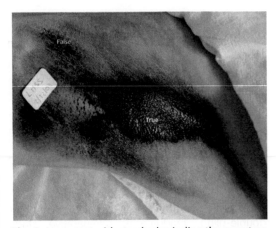

Fig. 1. In contact with starch plus iodine the sweat acquires a dark purple color (*center*), which is clearly visible. Normal areas need to be kept dry to avoid false reactions (*upper left quadrant*).

Therefore, the Minor test is mandatory to identify the actual affected area in a precise manner, so as to optimize the injection of the toxin and ensure effective treatment.

There are cases whereby sweating is excessive or is located outside the hairy area, as observed in **Fig. 2**. In such cases, if the BoNT treatment is confined to the terminal follicular area, the response will be unsatisfactory, as some regions will be left untreated. By contrast, when sweating is confined to small areas contained in the hairy region (**Figs. 3** and **4**), the treatment of the entire hair-bearing location implies in the use of an excessive and unnecessary amount of BoNT units. The distribution of the hyperhidrotic area frequently may assume different shapes, such as "M," "S," or "8," and the iodine-starch test will also highlight all of these situations (**Fig. 5**).

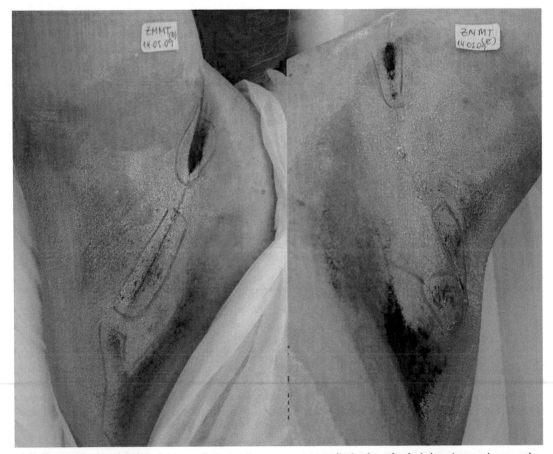

Fig. 2. In this female patient, the excessive sweating areas are not limited to the hair-bearing regions, and an effective botulinum toxin treatment cannot be achieved if precise localization is not delimited before the procedure.

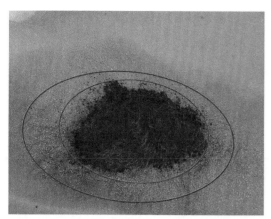

Fig. 3. In this male individual, the iodine-starch test shows that the hyperhidrotic region is smaller than the hairy area.

For iodine-sensitive patients, Ponceau red tincture is an alternative. When mixed with starch and in contact with sweat, this tincture develops a pinkish color.[39] For both techniques, the distribution and maximal perspiration sites must be recorded photographically for future comparison.

Another useful method for research trials, but time-consuming in daily practice (and thus not often applied), is gravimetric testing. The volume of produced sweat is measured over a fixed period of time under controlled conditions. First, the affected area is dried using absorbent tissue; then a previous weighed filter paper is applied and left in place for a certain period of time. The volume of produced sweat during this time interval is quantified by measuring the weight of the paper before and after contact. The evaluation period varies among investigators. One group prefers contact with the affected area for 1 minute,[20]

whereas other investigators prefer 5,[21,40] 10,[41] or 15 minutes.[42]

Use of the 2 aforementioned methods (gravimetry and Minor test) based on point counting using a transparent square-lattice grid was proposed by Bahmer and Sachse[41] as the Hyperhidrosis Area and Severity Index (HASI). One centimeter represents 1 point. After estimation of the sweating area, the volume of secretion weighed through gravimetry after 10 minutes is divided by the number of sites in the affected area. The HASI score is given in mg of sweat per cm^2 per minute. It is assumed hyperhidrosis is present if HASI values are greater than 1 mg/cm^2 per minute.

The quality of life of patients affected with focal idiopathic hyperhidrosis may be measured through several tests, the most frequently used being the Hyperhidrosis Disease Severity Scale.

INJECTION TECHNIQUE

After identifying and photographing the affected area, it has to be delimited with a marker pen or gentian violet. At this point it is possible to apply a local topical anesthetic, which will improve the patient's comfort during the procedure. If applied before, the anesthetic cream might impair the test.

The injection should be intradermal using a 30-gauge needle attached to the syringe (0.3- or 0.5-mL syringes, Ultrafine II 30-U or 50-U insulin syringes; Becton Dickinson, Franklin Lakes, NJ, USA), which eliminates the dead space between the needle and the syringe, and also the risk of expelling the needle during injection.

One study investigated whether the use of a 30-gauge rather than a 27-gauge needle influenced pain intensity in 38 patients treated with BoNT-A for axillary hyperhidrosis. The pain scores

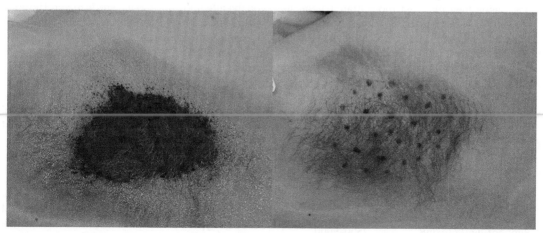

Fig. 4. In the same patient shown in **Fig. 3**, injection sites 1.5 cm apart are marked inside the delimited area.

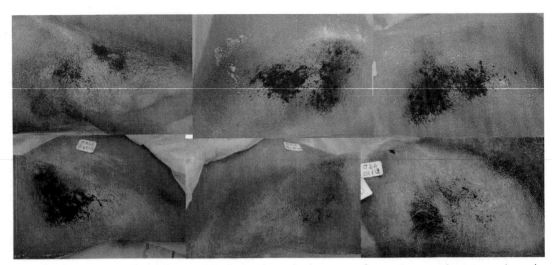

Fig. 5. Several underarms of different individuals where the locations of excessive sweating assume irregular, bizarre shapes.

recorded after the first 5 injections were significantly lower for the 30-gauge needle.[43]

The number of injections and the total dose depend on the involved surface area. Once injected, the toxin concentration will be higher at the central point, with a decreasing gradient along the peripheral areas.[37] The treatment goal is to create confluent overlapping anhidrotic halos to achieve an optimal outcome.[44] **Table 3** summarizes the usual BoNT doses for axillary hyperhidrosis as described in the literature.

Approximately 10 to 20 intradermal injections in 0.1- to 0.2-mL aliquots (total dose: 50–100 U OnaA) are used for each axilla, spaced 1 to 2 cm apart. Injections may also be performed in the superficial fat without adverse events or significant reduction in efficacy.

Most patients have excellent treatment results. The effects begin 2 to 4 days after injection and last approximately 6 to 9 months, although in some cases they may last more than 1 year. In the authors' experience, the longest successful outcomes are obtained when the excessive sweating location can be precisely delimited. Only when the patient could not sweat during iodine starch test the hair-bearing area is injected,

and in some of these cases, longer duration could not be achieved.

Figs. 6–8 show examples of short-term and long-term results after OnaA treatment of axillary hyperhidrosis.

Other techniques have been used as a variation of the traditional punctures. A device used for intralesional corticosteroid treatment of alopecia areata was described as an alternative method of BoNT application in axillary hyperhidrosis by means of a multi-injection round plate with 5 or 7 27-gauge needles. According to the investigators a rapid application in uniform and homogeneous manner was obtained, avoiding repeated punctures.[45]

A multiple-site marking grid has also been described, made of a flexible silicon sheet with holes punched out at a 1-cm distance (Exmoor Plastics Ltd, Taunton, UK). Once the excessive sweating area is defined, the grid is positioned on the affected area and the site is marked through the holes in the grid with a skin-marker pen. Jain[46] argues that this device saves time.

However, the use of these alternative techniques implies availability of the devices, whereas traditional injections only depend on easily available materials, in addition to well-trained professionals. **Box 1** provides a summary of practical information needed for successful BoNT treatment of excessive underarm sweating.

TRANSCUTANEOUS BOTULINUM TOXIN

There is a growing demand for the development of an effective, safe, and noninvasive treatment of axillary hyperhidrosis.[47] A means to deliver the toxin through the skin without needles or

Table 3	
Reported mean dose per axilla for each BoNT	
Toxin	Mean Dose (U)
OnabotulinumtoxinA	50–100
AbobotulinumtoxinA	100–300
IncobotulinumtoxinA	50
RimabotulinumtoxinB	2500–5000

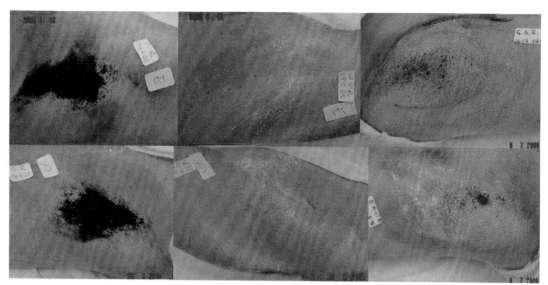

Fig. 6. A 28-year-old woman treated with 50 U of onabotulinumtoxinA (OnaA) per axilla. (*Upper and lower left*) Before treatment. (*Upper and lower central*) after 21 days. (*Upper and lower right*) After 15 months, when she returned for a new session.

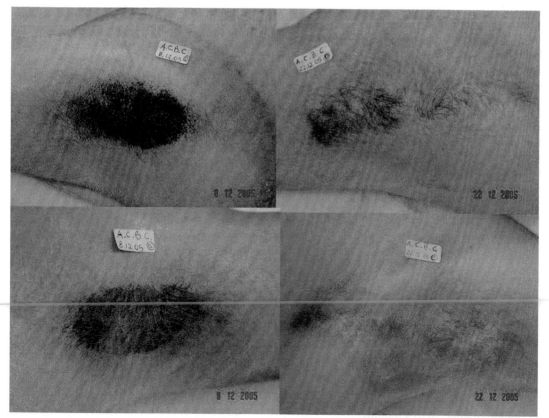

Fig. 7. A 29-year-old male patient, before (*left*) and after (*right*) his first treatment of 50 U OnaA per axilla.

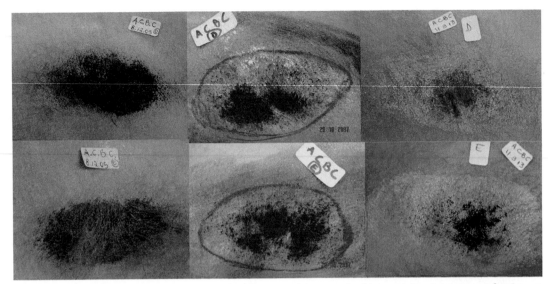

Fig. 8. The same patient shown in **Fig. 7**. He had been receiving regular biannual OnaA treatment for 8 years. (*Upper and lower left*) Before treatment. (*Upper and lower central*) Two years after his first treatment and just before the second. (*Upper and lower right*) After 4 biannual OnaA treatments. Note the long-term effect and possible reduction in the total extension of the affected area.

punctures has been recently tried, with promising results. However, BoNT directly applied to the skin is not absorbed because of its large molecular size.[48]

A small, controlled clinical trial investigated a novel proprietary transport peptide to deliver BoNT-A through the skin. Chow and Wilder-Smith[48] found a statistically significant reduction of sweat production in 12 cases of axillary hyperhidrosis using 200 U of OnaA reconstituted with saline admixed with the transport peptide. The duration of effect was not mentioned. This innovative method promises a revolution in the treatment of hyperhidrotic affected areas, and may also be useful in the future for other indications.

Box 1
Practical information for BoNT treatment of axillary hyperhidrosis

Always perform Minor test before applying BoNT-A

The test must be performed before any topical anesthesia

Highlight the area to be treated

Take photographs for future comparison

Distance between injection sites: 1 to 2 cm

Onset of action: 2 to 4 days

Duration of effect: 6 to 9 months

SUMMARY

BoNT has proved to be a safe and effective treatment for axillary hyperhidrosis. Although its pathophysiology remains controversial, the beneficial effect of type-A neuromodulators in temporarily inhibiting localized sweating supports a level A recommendation from evidence-based review.

REFERENCES

1. Doft MA, Kasten JL, Ascherman JA. Treatment of axillary hyperhidrosis with botulinum toxin: a single surgeon's experience with 53 consecutive patients. Aesthetic Plast Surg 2011;35:1079–86.
2. Glaser DA, Hebert AA, Pariser DM, et al. Primary focal hyperhidrosis: scope of the problem. Cutis 2007;79(5):5–17.
3. Hornberger J, Grimes K, Naumann M, et al. Recognition, diagnosis, and treatment of primary focal hyperhidrosis. J Am Acad Dermatol 2004;51:274–86.
4. Hamm H, Naumann MK, Kowalski JW, et al. Primary focal hyperhidrosis: disease characteristics and functional impairment. Dermatology 2006;212:343–53.
5. Sato K, Kang WH, Saga KT. Biology of sweat glands and their disorders I. Normal sweat gland function. J Am Acad Dermatol 1989;20:537–63.
6. Kreyden O, Scheidegger E. Anatomy of the sweat glands, pharmacology of botulinum toxin, and distinctive syndromes associated with hyperhidrosis. Clin Dermatol 2004;22:40–4.

7. Mota Juang J, Sotto MN. Anatomy and histology of sweat glands. In: Almeida AR, Hexsel DM, editors. Hyperhidrosis and botulinum toxin. São Paulo (Brazil): Edition of authors; 2004. p. 3–6.

8. Bovell DL, Clunes MT, Elder HY, et al. Ultrastructure of the hyperhidrotic eccrine sweat gland. Br J Dermatol 2001;145:298–301.

9. Bovell DL, MacDonald A, Meyer BA, et al. The secretory clear cell of the eccrine sweat gland as the probable source of excess sweat production in hyperhidrosis. Exp Dermatol 2011;20(12):1017–20.

10. Lindsay SL, Holmes S, Corbett AD, et al. Innervation and receptor profiles of the human apocrine (epitrichial) sweat gland: routes for intervention in bromhidrosis. Br J Dermatol 2008;159:653–60.

11. Atkins JL, Butler PE. Hyperhidrosis: a review of current management. Plast Reconstr Surg 2002;110: 222–8.

12. Sato K, Kang WT, Saga KT. Biology of sweat glands and their disorders II. Disorders of sweat gland function. J Am Acad Dermatol 1989;20:713–26.

13. Bovell D, Corbett A, Holmes S, et al. The absence of apoeccrine glands in the human axilla has disease pathogenetic implications, including axillary hyperhidrosis. Br J Dermatol 2007;156:1278–86.

14. Bechara F. Do we have apoeccrine sweat glands? Int J Cosmet Sci 2008;30:67–8.

15. Kalner IJ. Same-patient prospective comparison of Botox versus Dysport for treatment of primary axillary hyperhidrosis and review of literature. J Drugs Dermatol 2011;10(9):1013–5.

16. Trindade De Almeida AR, Secco LC, Carruthers A. Handling botulinum toxins: an updated literature review. Dermatol Surg 2011;37(11):1553–65.

17. Rosell K, Hymnelius K, Swartling C. Botulinum toxin type A and B improve quality of life in patients with axillary and palmar hyperhidrosis. Acta Derm Venereol 2013;93:335–9.

18. Lowe NJ, Glaser DA, Eadie N, et al. Botulinum toxin type A in the treatment of primary axillary hyperhidrosis: a 52-week multicenter double-blind, randomized, placebo-controlled study of efficacy and safety. J Am Acad Dermatol 2007;56(4):604–11.

19. Grunfeld A, Murray CA, Solish N. Botulinum toxin for hyperhidrosis: a review. Am J Clin Dermatol 2009; 10(2):87–102.

20. Heckmann M, Ceballos-Baumann AO, Plewig G. Botulinum toxin A for axillary hyperhidrosis (excessive sweating). N Engl J Med 2001;344(7):488–93.

21. Naumann M, Lowe NJ. Botulinum toxin type A in treatment of bilateral primary axillary hyperhidrosis: randomised, parallel group, double blind, placebo controlled trial. BMJ 2001;323(7):596–9.

22. Scamoni S, Valdatta L, Frigo C, et al. Treatment of primary axillary hyperhidrosis with botulinum toxin type A: our experience in 50 patients from 2007 to 2010. ISRN Dermatol 2012;2012:702714.

23. Lecouflet M, Leux C, Fenot M, et al. Duration of efficacy increases with the repetition of botulinum toxin A injections in primary axillary hyperhidrosis: a study in 83 patients. J Am Acad Dermatol 2013; 69(6):960–4.

24. Lakraj AA, Moghimi N, Jabbari B. Hyperhidrosis: anatomy, pathophysiology and treatment with emphasis on the role of botulinum toxins. Toxins (Basel) 2013;5:821–40.

25. Available at: http://www.fda.gov/Drugs/DrugSafety/PostmarketDrugSafetyInformationforPatientsand Providers/DrugSafetyInformationforHeathcareProfes sionals/ucm174949.htm. Accessed October 1, 2010.

26. Baumann L, Slezinger A, Halem M, et al. Pilot study of the safety and efficacy of MyoblocTM (botulinum toxin type B) for treatment of axillary hyperhidrosis. Int J Dermatol 2005;44:418–24.

27. Nelson L, Bachoo P, Holmes J. Botulinum toxin type B: a new therapy for axillary hyperhidrosis. Br J Plast Surg 2005;58:228–32.

28. Dressler D, Adib Saberi F, Benecke R. Botulinum toxin type B for treatment of axillar hyperhidrosis. J Neurol 2002;249(12):1729–32.

29. Frasson E, Brigo F, Acler M, et al. Botulinum toxin type A vs type B for axillary hyperhidrosis in a case series of patients observed for 6 months. Arch Dermatol 2011;147(1):122–3.

30. Naumann M, Dressler D, Hallett M, et al. Evidence-based review and assessment of botulinum neurotoxin for the treatment of secretory disorders. Toxicon 2013;67:141–52.

31. Talarico-Filho S, Mendonça DO, Nascimento M, et al. A double-blind, randomized, comparative study of two type A botulinum toxins in the treatment of primary axillary hyperhidrosis. Dermatol Surg 2007;33(1):44–50.

32. Dressler D. Comparing botox and xeomin for axillar hyperhidrosis. J Neural Transm 2010;117:317–9.

33. Gülec AT. Dilution of botulinum toxin A in lidocaine vs. in normal saline for the treatment of primary axillary hyperhidrosis: a double-blind, randomized, comparative preliminary study. J Eur Acad Dermatol Venereol 2012;26:314–8.

34. Vadoud-Seyedi J, Simonart T. Treatment of axillary hyperhidrosis with botulinum toxin type A reconstituted in lidocaine or in normal saline: a randomized, side-by-side, double-blind study. Br J Dermatol 2007;156:986–9.

35. Goodman G. Diffusion and Short-term efficacy of Botulinum toxin A after addition of hyaluronidase and its possible application for the treatment of axillary hyperhidrosis. Dermatol Surg 2003;29:533–8.

36. Cohen JL, Cohen G, Solish N, et al. Diagnosis, impact, and management of focal hyperhidrosis: treatment review including botulinum toxin therapy. Facial Plast Surg Clin North Am 2007;15: 17–30, v–vi.

37. Glogau R. Hyperhidrosis and botulinum toxin A: patient selection and techniques. Clin Dermatol 2004; 22:45–52.

38. Burks RI. Povidone-iodine solution in wound treatment. Phys Ther 1998;78(2):212–8.

39. Bushara KO, Park DM. Botulinum toxin and sweating [letter]. J Neurol Neurosurg Psychiatry 1994;54(11): 1437.

40. Hund M, Kinkelin I, Naumann M, et al. Definition of axillary hyperhidrosis by gravimetric assessment. Arch Dermatol 2002;138:539–41.

41. Bahmer F, Sachse M. Hyperhidrosis area and severity index [letter]. Dermatol Surg 2008;34: 1744–5.

42. Odderson IR. Long-term quantitative benefits of botulinum toxin A in the treatment of axillary hyperhidrosis. Dermatol Surg 2002;28:480–3.

43. Skiveren J, Larsen HN, Kjaerby E, et al. The influence of needle size on pain perception in patients treated with botulinum toxin A injections for axillary hyperhidrosis. Acta Derm Venereol 2011;91:72–4.

44. Klein AW. Complication, adverse reaction, and insights with the use of botulinum toxin. Dermatol Surg 2003;29:549–56.

45. Grimalt R, Moreno-Arias GA, Ferrando J. Multi-injection plate for botulinum toxin application in the treatment of axillary hyperhidrosis. Dermatol Surg 2001;27:543–4.

46. Jain S. A new multiple site marking grid for botulinum toxin application in the treatment of axillary hyperhidrosis. Br J Dermatol 2006;154:375–91.

47. Glogau RG. Topically applied botulinum toxin type A for the treatment of primary axillary hyperhidrosis: results of a randomized, blinded, vehicle-controlled study. Dermatol Surg 2007;33(1):S76–80.

48. Chow A, Wilder-Smith EP. Effect of transdermal botulinum toxin on sweat secretion in subjects with idiopathic palmar hyperhidrosis. Br J Dermatol 2009; 160(3):721–3.

Botulinum Neurotoxin Treatment of Palmar and Plantar Hyperhidrosis

Tessa Weinberg[a], Nowell Solish, MD, FRCPC[b],*,
Christian Murray, MD, FRCPC[b]

KEYWORDS

• Botulinum neurotoxin • Palmar plantar hyperhidrosis • Nerve blocks • Hypehidrosis

KEY POINTS

• Palmar and plantar hyperhidrosis is relatively common and can have severe psychological and medical consequences for those afflicted.
• A multitude of treatments exist but are often inadequate especially for those with significant disease; in these cases BoNT, in its various formulations, provides a reliable method for reducing the symptoms and improving QOL.
• Although the actual administration is relatively straightforward pain management is a crucial component that requires a mastery of several techniques.
• Patients have a high degree of satisfaction with BoNT treatment and are motivated to come back for repeat treatments, usually every 6 months.

INTRODUCTION AND OVERVIEW

Hyperhidrosis (HH) is an excessive sweating disorder that affects approximately 2.8% of the population in the United States,[1] likely with similar incidences in other countries.[2] It is commonly defined as sweating beyond what is expected for environmental conditions and thermoregulation with duration of more than 6 months.[3] Some have added specific diagnostic criteria, which are discussed later[4] and do apply to the palms and soles. A quantitative definition of HH as the production of more than 50 mg of sweat in one palm per minute has also been suggested for use in studies and when examining therapeutic intervention[5]; however, this fails to account for surface area. Clinically, sweating is considered excessive if it significantly interferes with daily life.

HH can be classified as primary or secondary and further as general or focal. Focal is further subclassified by anatomic area. Eccrine glands cover most of the body and have a density of approximately $60/cm^2$, except on the palms and soles where their density is at approximately $600/cm^2$.[6] It is thus not surprising that patients experience HH in areas of high eccrine density, such as the soles (30%) and palms (24%).[7] It should be noted that in primary focal HH, neither the number, density, nor size of eccrine glands are abnormal; rather, there is overactivity of the postganglionic sympathetic cholinergic fibers (sudomotor) innervating them.[8] This explains the effectiveness of botulinum neurotoxin (BoNT).

In clinical practice significantly more patients present with axillary than palmar HH and more with palmar than plantar HH.[9] In many cases individuals suffer with more than one site involved. Most patients who present with palmar HH have had the condition since childhood or early

[a] School of Medicine, Royal College of Surgeons of Ireland, 123 Street Stephen's Green, Dublin 2, Ireland;
[b] Division of Dermatology, Women's College Hospital, University of Toronto, 76 Grenville Street, Room 5142, Toronto, Ontario M5S 1B2, Canada
* Corresponding author. Division of Dermatology, Women's College Hospital, University of Toronto, 76 Grenville Street, Toronto, Ontario M5S 1B2, Canada.
E-mail address: n.solish@utoronto.ca

Dermatol Clin 32 (2014) 505–515
http://dx.doi.org/10.1016/j.det.2014.06.012
0733-8635/14/$ – see front matter © 2014 Elsevier Inc. All rights reserved.

adolescence with no known cause and report "sweaty palms" that cause them social embarrassment. The effects later in life are physical and emotional. Physically, the wetness may be bothersome enough that patients go to great lengths to avoid shaking peoples hands and frequently hide their hands in their pockets. Plantar HH may cause patients to frequently change their socks and slip in their shoes. HH is a well-established risk factor for cutaneous infection and eczematous dermatitis. Psychologically HH causes anxiety, emotional distress, embarrassment, and a markedly diminished quality of life (QOL).[3,4] Interestingly, a study by Lear and colleagues[7] suggested that spontaneous regression might occur over time because there is a low prevalence of the disorder in the elderly population.

Multiple modalities are available for treatment of primary focal HH, including topical medications, such as aluminum chloride[10]; oral medications, such as clonidine[3,11]; physical treatments, such iontophoresis[3,11]; injectable treatments, such as BoNT; and even surgical sympathectomy.[2,12]

In this article, the role of BoNT in the treatment of primary focal HH of the palms and soles is discussed.

PATIENT EVALUATION

A careful clinical history and focused physical are imperative. The first fact to establish is whether the patient has primary or secondary HH. There are many causes of secondary HH that have been well documented previously[13] and include febrile illness (ie, chronic infections), endocrine disorders (thyroid dysfunction), medication use (ie, antidepressants), and cancer (ie, pheochromcytoma). Secondary is more likely if the sweating is associated with other constitutional symptoms and is generalized in nature. If secondary HH is suspected the work-up should at minimum include a complete blood count, fasting glucose level, and thyroid function tests. Any suspected offending medications should be discontinued and if necessary appropriately substituted. Further investigations should be guided by elements of the history and the examination.

The generally accepted diagnostic criteria for HH in general and palmar-plantar specifically is excessive sweating that lasts at least 6 months without any obvious cause and has at least two of the following features: impairs daily activities, a bilateral and relatively symmetric pattern of sweating occurring at least once per week, an age of onset younger than 25 years, cessation of focal sweating during sleep, or positive family history.[4] Bilaterality is not a diagnostic criteria and it

should be noted that palmar HH can present unilaterally in 6% of cases.[4]

It is important to quantify the impact of HH on the patient's QOL.[14] This not only helps to decide on the need for and success of treatment but may also aide in obtaining insurance approval for treatment. The HH Disease Severity Scale (HDSS) is an easy tool for this (**Table 1**).

It is important to take a family history because there is evidence that primary HH is an autosomal-dominant trait with variable penetrance.[15,16]

MANAGEMENT GOALS AND STRATEGY

The goal of management is to improve the quality of the patient's life with acceptable risks. QOL studies have in general shown a significant improvement in the QOL after treatment of axillary,[17] for palmar and planter HH.[18]

Several methods have been used to measure the amount of palmar and plantar sweating before and after treatment. These include the evaporimeter,[19] persprint paper,[20] patient reports of the number of days of dryness,[21] digitized ninhydrine test,[22] gravimetry sweat production test,[23] the Minor iodine starch test,[24] and the HDSS. We clinically prefer the HDSS because it is easy and quick to administer and has been found[25] to be

Table 1 Hyperhidrosis Disease Severity Scale		
"How Would You Rate the Severity of Your Hyperhidrosis?" Patient Response	Score	Clinical Interpretation
1 My sweating is never noticeable and never interferes with my daily activities	1	Mild
2 My sweating is tolerable but sometimes interferes with my daily activities	2	Moderate
3 My sweating is barely tolerable and frequently interferes with my daily activities	3	Severe
4 My sweating is intolerable and always interferes with my daily activities	4	Very severe

a reliable diagnostic tool. It can also be used to monitor the effectiveness of treatment. Success may be considered a reduction in HDSS of 1 or more. Although a subjective test, it accurately reflects patient QOL, which is most relevant to patients.

The Canadian Hyperhidrosis Advisory Committee has made several treatment recommendations.[26] In review, the committee recommends topical aluminum chloride as a first-line option, in a concentration of 20% to 50% for treating mild focal or multifocal HH. For patients with moderate to severe HH, the committee recommends starting treatment with topical aluminum chloride and, if ineffective, trying iontophoresis or onabotulinumtoxinA (A/Ona) injections. Surgery should be reserved for patients who do not respond to less invasive interventions. Of note, endoscopic thoracic sympathectomy although established may have significant complications and deleterious side effects including compensatory HH. Surgery should be reserved for patients in whom less invasive treatments have proved ineffective and who understand the risks and benefits of the surgery.[2,12]

BoNT

There are four types of BoNTs approved by the Food and Drug Administration for clinical use in the United States: A/Ona (Botox; Allergan, Irvine, CA), A/Inco (Xeomin; Merz Pharmaceuticals, Greenboro, NC), abobotulinumtoxinA (A/Abo; Dysport; Medicis, Scottsdale, AZ), and rimabotulinumtoxinB (B/Rima, Myobloc; Solstice Neurosciences, Louisville, KY).

BoNTs block the release of acetylcholine and several other neurotransmitters from presynaptic vesicles by deactivating SNARE proteins. These toxins use different presynaptic proteins for their site of action. For instance, for A/Ona the protein is synaptin 25.

There are several important facts that must be considered before instituting therapy with BoNT. First, all four types of commercially available BoNT are considered pregnancy category C drugs and one should avoid injection in actively nursing women. Second, treatment of the palms and soles for primary focal HH is considered an off-label use of BoNT. Third, one must always screen for previous allergic reaction to BoNT. Fourth, one must be aware of the patient's current medication list because certain medications can theoretically alter the metabolism of neurotoxin, such as aminoglycoside antibacterials, cholinesterase inhibitors, and calcium channel antagonists. Finally, the use of BoNT can exacerbate some neuromuscular disorders, such as myasthenia gravis.

EVALUATION OF TREATMENT AND RECOMMENDATIONS

There are many different types of studies for BoNT treatment of palmar and plantar HH. The placebo-controlled evidence for palmar HH is reviewed in **Table 2**. There is one single-agent study each for A/Abo,[22] A/Ona,[23] and B/Rima.[25] These studies are small and of short duration; however, they do confirm the effectiveness of these products. This allows the conclusion that the evidence supports a Level B recommendation for BoNT-A and a Level C recommendation for BoNT-B for the treatment of palmar HH.[3,27] On further examination of the evidence one can conclude that there are insufficient data for the individual formulations, so each receives a Level U recommendation. The side effects were in the order of what is expected and are covered in more detail in the complications section.

The comparative effectiveness studies are interesting (see **Table 2**). In one study BoNT A/Ona and A/Abo at mean doses of 69 U and 284 U per palm, respectively, were compared.[24] The difference in doses is explained because the dose for A/Abo is usually relatively higher by a factor of 2.5 to 4. In a second the study 50 U of A/Ona and 100 U of A/Ona were compared,[28] and in a third study A/Ona and A/Inco were compared.[29] The Simonetta Moreau and coworkers[24] study showed no statistically significant difference at 1 month post-injection in the reduction in sweating between the A/Abo- and A/Ona-treated palms, although there was a tendency for greater efficacy of A/Abo. At 3 months, the reduced sweating persisted for the A/Abo- but not A/Ona-treated palms. The duration of effect ranged from 8 to 32 weeks with both agents (mean, 17 weeks for A/Abo and 18 weeks for A/Ona). In the study of two different doses of A/Ona, both doses reduced sweating in all patients at 2 months, with an evident anhidrotic effect at 6 months in one-third of both dose groups.[28] In the Campanati and coworkers study,[29] there were no differences in efficacy or side effects for the A/Ona and the A/Inco groups.

One can also see from **Table 2** that in a recent double-blind randomized study the effects of concentrations of A/Ona, A/Inca, A/About, and B/Rima were studied using the starch iodine test.[30] The optimal dose was 25 IU/mL for A/Ona and A/Inca, 100 U/mL for A/Abo, and 50 U/mL for B/Rima. They concluded that concentration is a critical factor when considering HH treatment.

In other studies efficacies of 80% to 90%, similar to that seen in axillary HH, have been described with the use of BoNT-A in the treatment of palmar HH[11] and this corresponds to our clinical

Table 2
Palmar hyperhidrosis: significant single agent and comparative studies

Reference	AAN Class	Design	N	Follow-Up	Agent	Dose	Results	Adverse Events
Placebo-Controled Studies								
Schnider et al,[22] 1997	II	R, DB, PC Within-group comparison	11	13 wk	A/Abo	120 MU/palm PCO contralateral palm	Sweat production dropped: 26%, 26%, and 31% at wk 3, 8, 13 (P<.001) and improvement in VAS 38%, 40% and 35% at wk 3, 8, 13, respectively (P = .002)	Minor, reversible weakness of handgrip lasting 2 and 5 wk In three patients.
Lowe et al,[23] 2002	II	R, DB, PC	19	28 d	A/Ona	100 U/palm, PCO in contralateral palm	Percentage change from baseline was greater A/On-treated palms at day 28 (P = .0037). Minor test confirmed results.	Finger tingling and numbness in one A/Ona patient. One patient bilateral hand pain.
Baumann et al,[25] 2005	II	R, DB, PC	20	120 d or event-driven until return of sweating	B/Rima	5000 U/palm or PCO	Patient assessed efficacy significant difference B/Rima through day 120. Physician assessment no difference at day 30. Mean duration of effect; 3.8 mo.	Transient dry mouth in 18. Transient muscle weakness in 12.
Comparative Studies								
Simonetta Moreau et al,[24] 2003	II	R, DB, active	8	6 mo	A/Ona or A/Abo	A/Ona, 69 U/palm, or A/Abo, 284 U	Decrease in mean PSA; 76.8% A/Abo (P = .002) vs 56.6% A/Ona (P = .003) at 1 mo. At 3 mo decrease in PSA was 69.4%, A/Abo (P = .008) and 48.8%. A/Ona (NS). Mean duration of benefit 17 wk A/Abo; 18 wk A/Ona.	Pinch weakness, two times more frequent in A/Abo than A/Inco.

Study	Phase	Design	N	Duration	Toxin	Dose	Results	Strength/Side effects
Saadia et al,[28] 2001	II	R, SB, comparison of two doses, intraindividual comparison	24	6 mo	A/Ona	50 U or 100 U/palm	Significant decrease in sweating within 1 mo. At 6 mo anhidrotic effect evident in both dose groups. Both doses effective at 1 mo and lasted 6 mo in low-dose, 5 mo in high-dose groups.	No difference in hand grip strength. Finger pinch strength decreased.
Campanati et al,[29] 2014	II	R, DB	25	6 mo	A/Ona and A/Inco	A/Ona, 100–150 U/palm, and A/Inco, 100–150 U in other palm	A/Ona and A/Inco equivalent short- and long-term effects.	No difference in muscle strength between A/Ona and A/Inco.
Rystedt et al,[30] 2013	II	R, DB	20	3 mo	A/Ona, A/Inco B/Rima, A/Abo	Varying doses	Optimal doses of A/Ona, A/Abdo, A/Inco, and B/Rima: 25 U/mL, 40 U/mL, 25 U/mL.	N/A

Abbreviations: A/Abo, abobotulinumtoxinA; AAN, American Academy of Neurology; A/Inco, incobotulinumA; A/Ona, onabotulinumtoxinA; B/Rima, rimabotulinumtoxinB; DB, double blind; MU, mouse unit; PC, placebo controlled; PCO, placebo; PSA, palm sweating area; R, randomized; SB, single blind; VAS, visual analog scale.

Adapted from Naumann M, Dressler D, Hallett M, et al. Evidence-based review and assessment of botulinum neurotoxin for the treatment of secretory disorders. Toxicon 2013;67:147; and Lakraj AA, Moghimi N, Jabari B. Hyperhidrosis: anatomy, patho physiology and treatment with emphasis on the role of botulinum toxins. Toxins (Basel) 2013;5:821–40.

experiences. However, response to therapy varies more than that seen in axillary HH.

There are no placebo-controlled studies for plantar HH. There are several small studies that show benefit of BoNT-A.[18,31–33] These studies show that BoNT is efficacious and well tolerated if appropriate pain management strategies are instituted.

BoNT has been used in combination with several agents, specifically aluminum chloride, for treatment of palmar and plantar HH.[10] However, this as in other combination studies is small and does not allow conclusions to be drawn. In our practice we find an efficacy of approximately 50%.

TREATMENT COMPLICATIONS

The most common side effects from injection of BoNT into the palms and soles are bruising and discomfort during and immediately after treatment. Significant bleeding is not usually an issue but it should be noted that reactive hyperemia might follow regional nerve blockade to the wrists, with increased oozing at each injection site. Frank hematomas are very uncommon. BoNT injections in the palm in general and those specifically can lead to weakness of the muscles of the hand and over time may lead to atrophy (see **Table 2**, multiples studies). Weakness is quite common (see **Table 2**), more frequent with higher doses of the agent,[28] and at least in one study more frequent with BoNT A/abo than A/Ona. Although the weakness is usually of short duration, in one study it lasted 6 months.[28] Of note, one study showed the HH increased after treatment of the palms with BoNT injections[32]; however, this has not been our experience.

Palmar injections can be complicated by adverse events related to regional nerve blocks, such as inadvertent vascular puncture, impaired hand dexterity, and neuropathy from repeated nerve injuries, as reported by several authors.[34]

PROCEDURE FOR ADMINISTRATION OF BONT
BoNT Dilution

Dilution is an issue that one must contend with because there are many potential dilutions for BoNT. There is no consensus on the amount of dilution to use. One author has suggested that the optimal dilution of A/Ona is 25 U/mL.[30] We find that for palmar and plantar injections, reconstitution of one vial of Botox (100 units) with 3 mL of bacteriostatic preserved saline results in a manageable dilution (33 U/mL) for injection. With the 3-mL dilution, each 0.1 mL results in 3.3 IU of

Botox. To prevent toxin wastage in the vial and to avoid blunting the needle we recommend removing the bottle stopper. To avoid toxin wastage in the syringe we always use hubless syringes. It is important also not to let the needle touch the bottom of the vial because it blunts the needle. If using A/Abo Dysport for HH (300 units per vial) we recommend diluting with 3 mL of bacteriostatic preserved saline, which gives a final dilution of 10 U per 0.1 mL.

Multiple Needles for Injection

Given that palmar and plantar skin is very thick, needles dull quickly after serial injection. We therefore draw up the A/Ona Botox 100 U into six 0.5-mL syringes (B&D Ultra-Fine II 30-gauge hubless insulin needle syringes; Becton-Dickinson, Franklin Lakes, NJ). This ensures the needles are changed regularly and makes it easier to inject the fluid in the thick dermis.

Iodine Starch Test

The Minor iodine-starch test (**Figs. 1** and **2**) can be used to estimate the surface area of involvement that requires treatment. We have found this test of limited value initially, in that it tends to show involvement of the entire palm or sole and that it poorly estimates the amount of sweating. It is of significant value in follow-up to help delineate any missed areas (see **Fig. 2**). For most patients, we advocate marking both the hands and feet in a gridlike pattern with a pen.

Injection Pain Reduction

Injection pain is a very significant factor in the treatment of patients with palmar or plantar HH and pain is likely a significant factor in compliance. Many techniques have been proposed to reduce the pain. These include needle-free anesthesia[35]; ice[36]; skin cooling devices, such as those made by Zimmer; vibration analgesia[37];

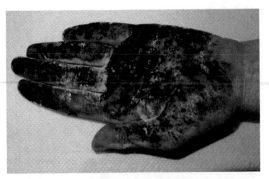

Fig. 1. Starch iodine test of a palm before treatment.

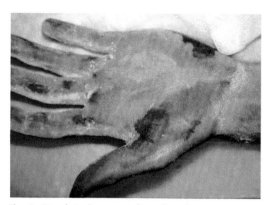

Fig. 2. Starch iodine test of a palm after treatment.

pocketed microneedles[38]; modified Bier blocks[39]; and nerve blocks.[40] These methods can be used in combination routinely or when a nerve block is incomplete. In our practice, we advise the use of either ice, a high-intensity vibration device (eg, AcuVibe, Poway, CA), or nerve blocks alone or in combination adjacent to each injection site to overstimulate nerve fibers.

Ice alone is used frequently in our HH clinic. Ice cubes held with gauze (or frozen with gauze on the outside) must be held on the skin for approximately 10 seconds before injection.[36] The ice is then moved to the next location while the injection is taking place. Ice is preferred over freezer packs because ice maintains a constant temperature. An absorbent pad under the hand is recommended to help with the melting ice. When using a cooling device for pain control on the palms, be careful to avoid freezing the BoNT solution in the needle when injecting.

Nerve Blocks

Nerve blocks are also used frequently by us and others[40] with success. Nerve blocks do have several disadvantages. These include the issues that there is a steep learning curve, that they are very user dependent, that nerve injury is a significant risk, that the patients spend a long time in the office, and that the patients generally cannot drive themselves home.

For the palms, median and ulnar nerve blocks are required (**Fig. 3**). It is imperative to know the relevant anatomy (**Fig. 4**). To perform a median nerve block, locate the palmaris longus tendon and the flexor carpi radialis tendon just proximal to the proximal wrist crease. The best way to accentuate these tendons is to ask the patient to make a fist and then to ask them to resist you pushing the wrist into extension. We then insert the needle just proximal to the proximal wrist

crease between the palmaris longus and flexor carpi radialis tendons. We usually inject 2 mL of 1% lidocaine. We inject 0.3 mL above the fascia to get the palmar cutaneous nerve and 1.7 mL below the fascia for the main nerve. It is imperative to warn the patient that if they feel any unusual pain, numbness, tingling, and "shocks" during the injection that they should tell you immediately because this may signify intraneural injection.

For the ulnar nerve block, we identify the flexor carpi ulnaris tendon at the proximal wrist crease. To find the flexor carpi ulnaris tendon, we ask the patient to make a fist, then ulnarly deviate the wrist, and finally resist you pushing the wrist into extension.

We usually inject 2 mL of 1% lidocaine just radial to flexor carpi ulnaris at the proximal wrist crease. Once again we inject 0.3 mL above the fascia to get the dorsal sensory branch of the ulnar nerve and 1.7 mL below the fascia to get the main nerve. It is important to watch for symptoms of intraneural injection. In each case one should always withdraw to ensure that the needle tip is not intravascular.

For plantar injections, sural nerve and posterior tibial nerve blocks are needed.[13] A sural nerve block anesthetizes the fifth toe and lateral side of the sole. It requires injection of 3 to 5 mL of 1% lidocaine between the lateral malleolus and the Achilles tendon. A posterior tibial nerve block anesthetizes the heel and middle of the sole of the foot. For this nerve block, palpate the posterior tibial artery near the medial malleolus. The nerve is lateral to the artery. Inject 5 mL of 1% lidocaine in the groove between the medial malleolus and the Achilles tendon. Wait 15 minutes for regional nerve blocks to take full effect. Regional nerve blocks may be incomplete despite several attempts. In these cases we add ice or the AcuVibe.

Treatment Area

The hands and feet are marked in a gridlike pattern (**Figs. 5** and **6**). Each injection point is spaced 1- to 1.5-cm apart because it is likely less diffusion occurs on the palms and soles compared with other body sites. With experience, the grid pattern becomes second nature to the injector and the sterile pen markings are not required.

The BoNT should ideally be placed at the junction of the dermis and the subcutaneous tissue because this corresponds to the location of the eccrine glands. However, given the likelihood of significant muscle weakness (see **Table 2**) with a subcutaneous injection our preference is to place the injections intradermal, which thus limits

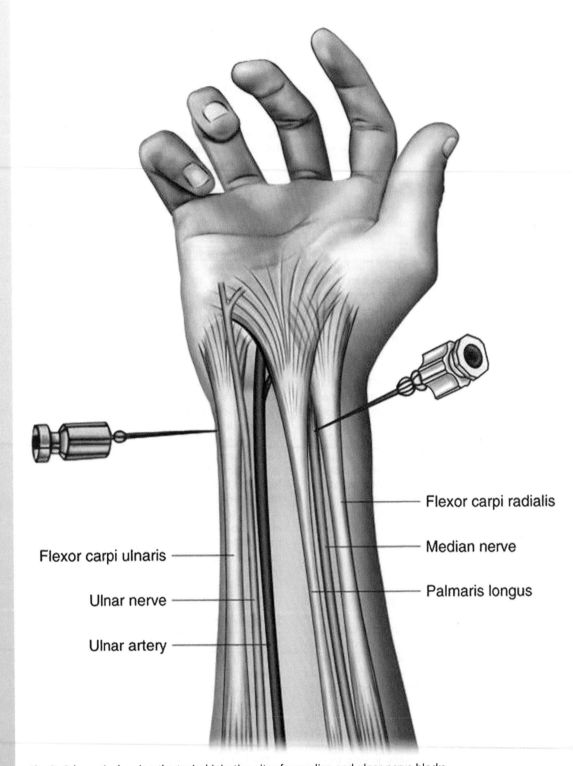

Fig. 3. Schematic showing the typical injection sites for median and ulnar nerve blocks.

diffusion of the product into the muscles. This is more important in the hands than the feet because there is less subcutaneous tissue in the hands and weakness in the hands would be more noticeable.

Weakness usually presents with complaints, such as difficulty using a key or activities that require grip strength. One should note that it is common to see a small zone of blanching and uncommon

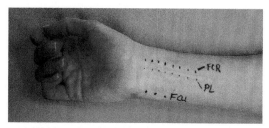

Fig. 4. Forearm surface anatomy showing the tendons of flexor carpi ulnaris (FCU), flexor carpi radialis (FCR), and palmaris longus (PL).

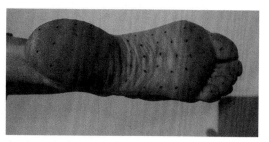

Fig. 6. Typical injection grid for the foot.

to see a wheel around each injection point on the palms and soles.

Injection Dose

The optimal dosing for palms and feet is uncertain because of a paucity of studies. Some authors recommend a range from 50 to 100 U for A/Ona and 100 to 240 U of Abo/A BoNT per hand (see **Table 2**). The size of the hand helps to determine the final dose. Two to thee units should be used for each injection site. Muscle weakness in the hand is an issue and may be dose dependent so we recommend starting with 50 U A/Ona Botox per hand then reassessing the first-time patient at 1 month. Injections have been shown to last about 6 months[13,32] and are thus typically repeated every 6 months.

Injection Technique

The intradermal injection technique required in the palms and soles tends to result in backflow, which can manifest as leaking out of the injection site. There are several injection techniques to minimize this. They include injecting with the bevel down, maximal acute angling of the needle to the skin surface, injecting slowly over 1 to 2 seconds to allow time for normalization of pressure, pausing for 1 second after

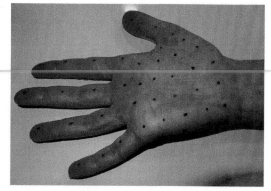

Fig. 5. Typical injection grid for the palm.

injection is complete before withdrawing the needle, and making sure there are no air bubbles in the syringe.[34,41]

Patient Monitoring and Followup

Patients are monitored in the office for signs and symptoms of adverse events and encouraged to report any that occur following treatments and between follow-up visits. We counsel patients that they will begin to notice a difference in 7 to 10 days. We recommend follow-up every 5 months in treatment-naive patients and every 6 to 7 months in patients treated on a regular basis. We routinely call patients within 2 weeks of treatment to confirm that they have noted a decrease in symptoms.

For patients who are in professions that require fine hand movement and strength, we recommend first treating the nondominant hand and then the dominant hand at a later visit after further discussion with the patient.

SUMMARY

Palmar and plantar HH is relatively common and can have severe psychological and medical consequences for those afflicted. A multitude of treatments exist but are often inadequate especially for those with significant disease. In these cases BoNT, in its various formulations, provides a reliable method for reducing the symptoms and improving the QOL. Most of the studies have been done for Botox A/Ona and show significant efficacy. Although the actual administration is relatively straightforward, pain management is a crucial component that requires a mastery of several techniques. Patients have a high degree of satisfaction with BoNT treatment and are motivated to come back for repeat treatments, usually every 6 months.

REFERENCES

1. Strutton DR, Kowalski JW, Glaser DA, et al. US prevalence of hyperhidrosis and impact on

individuals with axillary hyperhidrosis: results from a national survey. J Am Acad Dermatol 2004; 51(2):241–8.

2. Lin TS, Fang HY. Transthoracic endoscopic sympathectomy in the treatment of palmar hyperhidrosis—with emphasis on perioperative management (1360 case analyses). Surg Neurol 1999;52:453–7.

3. Lakraj AA, Moghimi N, Jabari B. Hyperhidrosis: anatomy, pathophysiology and treatment with emphasis on the role of botulinum toxins. Toxins (Basel) 2013;5:821–40.

4. Hornberger J, Grimes K, Naumann M. Recognition, diagnosis, and treatment of primary focal hyperhidrosis. J Am Acad Dermatol 2004;51:274–8.

5. Naumann MK, Hamm J, Lowe NJ. Effect of botulinum toxin type A on quality of life measures in patients with excessive maxillary sweating: a randomized controlled trial. Br J Dermatol 2002;147: 1218–26.

6. Sato K. The physiology, pharmacology and biochemistry of the eccrine sweat gland. Rev Physiol Biochem Pharmacol 1997;79:51–131.

7. Lear W, Kessler E, Solish N. An epidemiological study of hyperhidrosis. Dermatol Surg 2007;33:S69–75.

8. Manca D, Valls-Sole J, Callejas MA. Excitability recovery curve of the sympathetic skin response in healthy volunteers and patients with palmar hyperhidrosis. Clin Neurophysiol 2000;111:1767–70.

9. Glaser DA, Herbert AA, Pariser DM, et al. Palmar and plantar hyperhidrosis: best practice recommendations and special considerations. Cutis 2007;79(5):18–28.

10. Wooley-Loyd H, Valins W. Aluminum chloride hexahydrate in a salicylic acid gel base: a case series of combination therapy with botulinum toxin type A for moderate to severe hyperhidrosis. Cutis 2011; 88:43–5.

11. Walling HW, Swick BL. Treatment options for hyperhidrosis. Am J Clin Dermatol 2011;12(5):285–95.

12. Lewis DR, Irvine CD, Smith FC, et al. Sympathetic skin response and patient satisfaction on long-term follow-up after thoracoscopic sympathectomy for hyperhidrosis. Eur J Endo Vasc Surg 1998;15(3): 239–43.

13. Grunfeld A, Murray CA, Solish N. Botulinum toxin for hyperhidrosis: a review. Am J Clin Dermatol 2009; 10(2):87–102.

14. Hamm H, Naumann M, Kowalski JW, et al. Primary focal hyperhidrosis: disease characteristics and functional impairment. Dermatology 2006;212:343–53.

15. Haider A, Solish N. Focal hyperhidrosis: diagnosis and management. CMAJ 2005;172(1):69–75.

16. Kaufmann H, Saadia D, Polin C. Primary hyperhidrosis: evidence for autosomal dominant inheritance. Clin Auton Res 2003;13(2):96–8.

17. Solish N, Benohanian A, Kowalski JW, Canadian Dermatology Study Group on Health-Related Quality of Life in Primary Axillary Hyperhidrosis. Prospective open-label study of botulinum toxin type A in patients with axillary hyperhidrosis: effects on functional impairment and quality of life. Dermatol Surg 2005;31:405–13.

18. Campanati A, Bernardino ML, Gesuita R, et al. Plantar focal idiopathic hyperhidrosis and botulinum toxin: a pilot study. Eur J Dermatol 2007;17(1):52–4.

19. Goh CL. Aluminum chloride hexahydrate versus palmar hyperhidrosis. Evaporimeter assessment. Int J Dermatol 1990;29(5):368–70.

20. Akins DL, Meisenheimer JL, Dobson RL. Efficacy of the drionic unit in the treatment of hyperhidrosis. J Am Acad Dermatol 1987;16(4):828–32.

21. Dolianitis C, Scarff CE, Kelly J, et al. Iontophoresis with glycopyrrolate for the treatment of palmoplantar hyperhidrosis. Australas J Dermatol 2004;45(4):208–12.

22. Schnider P, Binder M, Auff E, et al. Double-blind trial of botulinum A toxin for the treatment of focal hyperhidrosis of the palms. Br J Dermatol 1997; 136:548–52.

23. Lowe NJ, Yamauchi PS, Lask GP, et al. Efficacy and safety of botulinum toxin type a in the treatment of palmar hyperhidrosis: a double-blind, randomized, placebo-controlled study. Dermatol Surg 2002;28: 822–7.

24. Simonetta Moreau M, Cauhepe C, Magues JP, et al. A double-blind, randomized, comparative study of dysport vs botox in primary palmar hyperhidrosis. Br J Dermatol 2003;149:1041–5.

25. Baumann L, Slezinger A, Halem M, et al. A double-blind, randomized, placebo-controlled pilot study of the safety and efficacy of myobloc (botulinum toxin type B) for the treatment of palmar hyperhidrosis. Dermatol Surg 2005;31:263–70.

26. Solish N, Bertucci V, Dansereau A. A comprehensive approach to the recognition, diagnosis, and severity-based treatment of focal hyperhidrosis: recommendations of the Canadian Hyperhidrosis Advisory Committee. Dermatol Surg 2007;33(8):908–23.

27. Naumann M, Dressler D, Hallett M, et al. Evidence-based review and assessment of botulinum neurotoxin for the treatment of secretory disorders. Toxicon 2013;67:141–52.

28. Saadia D, Voustianiouk A, Wang AK, et al. Botulinum toxin type A in primary palmar hyperhidrosis: randomized, single-blind, two-dose study. Neurology 2001;57:2095–9.

29. Campanati A, Giuliodori K, Martina E, et al. Onabotulinumtoxin type A (Botox) versus incobotulinumtoxin type A (Xeomin) in the treatment of focal idiopathic palmar hyperhidrosis: results of a comparative double-blind clinical trial. J Neural Transm 2014; 121(1):21–6.

30. Rystedt A, Karlqvist M, Bertilson M, et al. Effect botulinum toxin concentration on reduction of sweating: a randomised, double blind study. Acta Derm Venereol 2013;93:674–8.

31. Benohanian A. Treatment of recalcitrant plantar hyperhidrosis with type-A botulinum toxin injections and aluminum chloride in salicylic acid gel. Dermatol Online J 2008;14(2):5.

32. Gregoriou S, Rigopoulos D, Makris M, et al. Effects of botulinum toxin therapy for palmar hyperhidrosis in plantar sweat production. Dermatol Surg 2010; 36:496–8.

33. Tracey C, Vlahovic TC, Dunn SP, et al. Injectable botulinum toxin as a treatment for plantar hyperhidrosis. A case study. J Am Podiatr Med Assoc 2008;98(2): 156–9.

34. Fujita M, Mann T, Mann O, et al. Surgical pearl: use of nerve blocks for botulinum toxin treatment of palmar-plantar hyperhidrosis. J Am Acad Dermatol 2001;45:587–9.

35. Benohanian A. Needle-free anaesthesia prior to botulinum toxin type A injection treatment of palmar and plantar hyperhidrosis. Br J Dermatol 2007;156(3): 593–6.

36. Smith K. Ice minimizes discomfort associated with injection of botulinum toxin type A for the treatment of palmar and plantar hyperhidrosis. Dermatol Surg 2007;33:S88–91.

37. Moraru E, Auff E. Hyperhidrosis of the palms and soles. Curr Probl Dermatol 2002;30:156–69.

38. Torrisi BM, Zarnitsyn V, Prausnitz MR, et al. Pocketed microneedles for rapid delivery of a liquid-state botulinum toxin A formulation into human skin. J Control Release 2013;165:146–52.

39. Solomon P. Modified bier block anesthetic technique is safe for office use for botulinum a toxin treatment of palmar hyperhidrosis. Dermatol Online J 2007; 13(3):6.

40. Hayton MJ, Stanley JK, Lowe NJ. A review of peripheral nerve blockade as local anaesthesia in the treatment of palmar hyperhidrosis. Br J Dermatol 2003; 149:447–51.

41. Murray CA, Cohen JL, Solish N. Treatment of focal hyperhidrosis. J Cutan Med Surg 2007;11:67–77.

Botulinum Toxin for Hyperhidrosis of Areas Other than the Axillae and Palms/Soles

Dee Anna Glaser, MD*, Timur A. Galperin, DO

KEYWORDS

- Inguinal • Submammary • Facial • Compensatory • Amputee hyperhidrosis • Botulinum toxin

KEY POINTS

- Hyperhidrosis can affect many different areas of the body. Identifying and localizing the specific hyperhidrotic area with starch-iodine testing is important.
- Botulinum neurotoxin-A is an effective and safe treatment option for hyperhidrotic areas of the body.
- Patients should be counseled about their expectations with treatment.
- Injections should be placed at the dermal-subcutaneous junction.
- The dosing and the duration of effect of botulinum toxin are variable, and depend on the location and size of the involved area.

INTRODUCTION

Primary hyperhidrosis (HH) commonly affects the axillae, palms, and soles, but may occur on many body sites including the scalp, face, submammary regions, and groin (Table 1).[1,2] There are limited treatment options available for HH of areas other than the axillae and palms/soles. Although topical treatments are usually considered the first-line therapy, botulinum neurotoxin-A (BoNT-A) is an effective and safe treatment option for most hyperhidrotic areas of the body. This article focuses on BoNT-A treatment of hyperhidrosis of areas other than the axillae and palms/soles. Areas that are commonly affected, such as the face and groin, and less common areas like the submammary region and gluteal cleft, are discussed. Frey syndrome, compensatory sweating, and postamputation stump hyperhidrosis are also discussed.

PATIENT EVALUATION OVERVIEW

A thorough HH history and review of symptoms should be obtained from the patient, including age of onset of HH, location and symmetry of sweating, aggravating/alleviating factors, prior treatments for HH, family history of HH, and current medications that may exacerbate the condition. A physical examination should also be performed to help rule out a possible secondary cause of HH and to localize the affected area. A starch-iodine test is then performed to identify the dimensions of the involved area for treatment.

Disclosure: D.A. Glaser has served as advisor for Allergan, Galderma, Miramar Labs, and Unilever. She has been an investigator and received research grants from Allergan, Miramar Labs, and Ulthera. T.A. Galperin has nothing to disclose.
Department of Dermatology, Saint Louis University School of Medicine, 1402 South Grand Boulevard-ABI, St Louis, MO 63104, USA
* Corresponding author.
E-mail address: glasermd@slu.edu

Dermatol Clin 32 (2014) 517–525
http://dx.doi.org/10.1016/j.det.2014.06.001
0733-8635/14/$ – see front matter © 2014 Elsevier Inc. All rights reserved.

Table 1
Most common body sites of hyperhidrosis in a North American population

Body Site	Percentage of Patients
Axilla	73.0
Palms	45.9
Soles	41.1
Face or scalp	22.8
Groin	9.3
Other[a]	9.6

[a] Other includes sites such as the chest, back, abdomen, arms, or legs.

Data from Lear W, Kessler E, Solish N, et al. An epidemiological study of hyperhidrosis. Dermatol Surg 2007;33(s1): S69–75.

The Minor starch-iodine test is an inexpensive and simple procedure commonly used to localize focal areas of sweating. The starch-iodine test does not correspond with the severity of disease, and it may not be possible to illicit a response at every visit. Before performing this test, every patient should be asked about allergies to iodine. To perform the Minor starch-iodine test, the affected area is first thoroughly dried, then a solution of iodine in castor oil is brushed onto the skin and allowed to dry. In addition, corn starch powder is sprinkled on top, and the area is observed for a few minutes. A modified starch-iodine test is more commonly used in clinical practice and generally a povidone-iodine–based surgical preparation, such as Betadine, is used instead of the iodine-castor oil solution. Purple-black dots develop when sweat interacts with the starch and iodine (**Fig. 1**). The treating practitioner can then use a marking pen to create evenly spaced injection markings as a template for BoNT-A injections.

MANAGEMENT GOALS AND BOTULINUM TOXIN PREPARATION

The goals of BoNT-A therapy are to provide a long-lasting reduction in excess sweating, with the smallest effective amount of BoNT-A, and with minimal side effects. It is important to manage patient expectations so that there is an understanding that the goal is improvement in excess sweating, but that complete anhidrosis is rarely achieved. Risks of the procedure should be reviewed and an informed consent obtained. The authors have patients, or their representatives, review and sign a consent form before each treatment session. Most patients undergo repeated treatments over the years, and an untoward effect could occur with any injection session.

The only BoNT-A approved by the US Food and Drug Administration for axillary hyperhidrosis is onabotulinumtoxin-A (ona-BoNT-A; Botox [Allergan, Irvine, CA]), and it is the most common BoNT-A used off-label for hyperhidrosis of all involved areas. Abobotulinumtoxin-A (abo-BoNT-A; Dysport [Ipsen Ltd, Slough, Berkshire, UK]) has also been used effectively for hyperhidrosis. Ona-BoNT-A and abo-BoNT-A are not bioequivalent, and there is no consensus on the ideal conversion factor between these two preparations. The ratio of efficacy in axillary and palmar hyperhidrosis ranges from 1:1.5 to 1:3 for ona-BoNT-A/abo-BoNT-A,[3–5] and is unknown for other forms of hyperhidrosis. Incobotulinumtoxin-A (Xeomin, Merz Pharmaceuticals, Frankfurt, Germany) is a newer BoNT-A that has been shown to be effective in axillary and palmar hyperhidrosis in several studies,[6] and has been shown to be of equal efficacy to ona-BoNT-A for palmar hyperhidrosis in a single study.[7] We have the most experience with ona-BoNT-A for hyperhidrosis, and typically use it to treat patients with hyperhidrosis.

For axillary HH, the recommended reconstitution of ona-BoNT-A is with 4.0 mL of 0.9% nonpreserved saline, although we prefer to use preserved saline, which does not affect ona-BoNT-A efficacy.[2] The dilution volume of 4.0 mL allows for 2.5 units of ona-BoNT-A to be injected in a volume of 0.1 mL. Other volumes of diluent can be used for toxin reconstitution. In general, the more dilute the solution, the more diffusion of the drug that occurs, and this should be taken into consideration.[8] Injections are usually performed with a 1-mL Luer-Lock syringe and 30-gauge 12.5-mm needle. The drug should be placed at the dermal-subcutaneous junction, which is where the sweat glands reside, and this injection depth also minimizes the risk of diffusion to deeper muscles. In general, the needle is inserted into the skin at an oblique angle to maintain the superficial placement of the drug, and to minimize any loss of the botulinum solution. A small amount of blanching may be seen when BoNT-A is injected properly into the dermis.[2]

CRANIOFACIAL HYPERHIDROSIS

Primary hyperhidrosis of the scalp most commonly displays one of 4 patterns: the forehead; a band-like distribution around the scalp, known as the ophiasis pattern; a combination of the forehead and ophiasis scalp; or the entire scalp and forehead.[2] Less commonly involved areas include the upper lip, cheeks, nose, and chin. Several areas can be involved simultaneously.[2] With the exception of Frey syndrome, primary HH is not

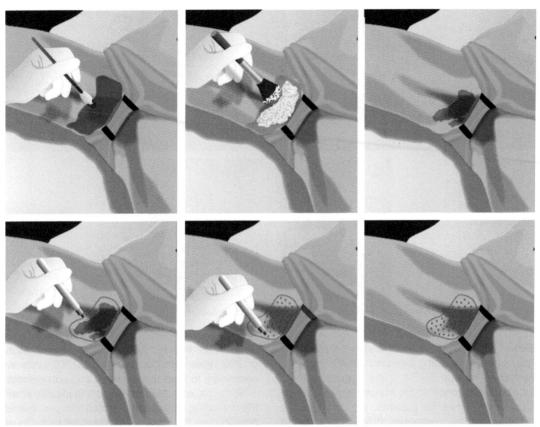

Fig. 1. Proper sequence for the Minor starch-iodine test, and marking the area for injection. First, the hyperhidrotic area is dried and an iodine solution is painted on and allowed to dry. Corn starch is then sprinkled on the area and allowed to sit for several minutes. Purple-black dots develop when sweat interacts with the starch and iodine. The treating practitioner can then use a marking pen to create evenly spaced injection markings as a template for BoNT-A injections. (*Courtesy of* Albert Ganss, International Hyperhidrosis Society, Quakertown, PA; with permission.)

usually unilateral, and patients presenting with unilateral involvement should be worked up for possible neurologic disease.[2] The Minor starch-iodine test helps to identify the specific distribution of sweating on the forehead and other areas of the face (**Fig. 2**) but is not practical for scalp involvement, unless the patient is bald. The importance of performing a starch-iodine test is highlighted in **Fig. 2C**, which shows involvement of the nasal ala, an uncommonly involved area of the nose.

BoNT-A treatment of facial HH should be carefully performed, because of the numerous muscles in the treatment areas. Even with properly placed injections, there is a possibility of having muscle weakness around the injection site, which may cause temporary functional and/or cosmetic irregularity.[2] The total amount of ona-BoNT-A, and the number of intradermal injection sites, varies with the location and pattern of sweating. Treatment of facial HH with abo-BoNT-A is also effective, although abo-BoNT-A has a greater

area of diffusion compared with ona-BoNT-A,[9] and there may be a greater potential of adverse events within this area.[9] With the exception of the forehead, there is a paucity of published literature on BoNT-A treatment of facial and scalp hyperhidrosis.

The average total dose of Botox for the forehead is approximately 40 units, with a range of 33 to 100 units.[2] For the forehead, 2 to 3 units of Botox per injection site, spaced at regular 1-cm to 2-cm intervals should be delivered to the dermal-subcutaneous junction. This dose ensures confluence of the medication, and minimizes diffusion into the muscles.[2] Avoiding the 1-cm to 2-cm area above the eyebrows may be needed to avoid brow ptosis, which is especially important in individuals with preexisting brow ptosis. Some patients may need to have the most inferior portion of their forehead treated to provide maximum improvement of their sweating, but they need to be warned of potential eyebrow and eyelid ptosis,

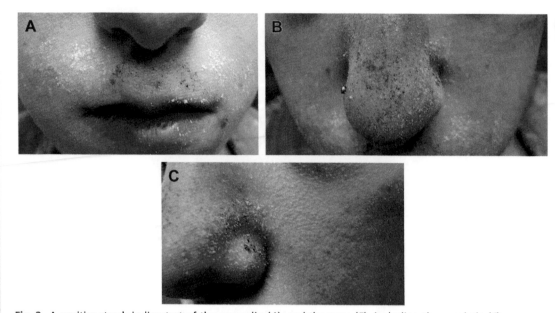

Fig. 2. A positive starch-iodine test of the upper lip (A), and the nose (B), including the nasal ala (C).

both of which are temporary and self-limited.[2] In most patients, treating the area above and into the hairline is required.[2] It is the authors' experience that injections into the frontal hairline provide superior outcomes for patients. We usually carry the injections approximately 2 to 4 cm into the hair-bearing scalp or based on the starch-iodine test if the patient is bald. **Fig. 3** shows an example of the proper injection technique for the forehead. Most commonly it is our practice to use 100 units of ona-BoNT-A for this area.

When treating the ophiasis pattern of scalp hyperhidrosis, we commonly inject 100 units of ona-BoNT-A. Approximately 2.5 units are injected at 2-cm intervals. When the entire scalp is treated (excluding the forehead), ∼2.5 units of ona-

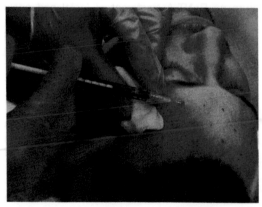

Fig. 3. Botulinum toxin injection technique into the forehead. (*Courtesy of* Albert Ganss, International Hyperhidrosis Society, Quakertown, PA; with permission.)

BoNT-A are injected at 2-cm intervals, for a total of 200 units.[10] In our experience, 300 units are necessary to treat the forehead and entire scalp.

Some patients may not be able to identify where the sweating originates, because it can quickly spread over the scalp. It is important to try to get the patient to pinpoint the location to help reduce the numbers of units needed. If a subunit of the scalp is not treated and the patient discovers that it is affected, the physician can treat the missed area at a future appointment. It is difficult to perform a starch-iodine test in the hair-bearing scalp. We sometimes ask patients to do some light exercise or walking in the office to try to elicit a sweat response such that we can determine the areas that need to be treated and estimate the amount of botulinum toxin needed.

Botulinum toxin-A can be safely and effectively administered for nasal HH. A dose of 1 to 2 units per injection spaced every 0.5 to 1.0 cm, for a total dose of 10 to 20 units of ona-BoNT-A, is usually required.[11,12] Take care to avoid the lacrimal system and the nasal muscles when injecting at the lateral nasal wall, keeping injections as medial as possible. Very small aliquots should be injected superficially to help avoid muscle effects. Patients should be warned of a drooping of the upper lip and an inability to flare the nostrils. The latter can decrease air intake through the nostrils with heavy exercise.

Upper lip hyperhidrosis can been treated effectively with ∼1 unit of ona-BoNT-A per injection, spaced at 0.5-cm intervals,[13] or with 2 units per injection, spaced at 1 cm.[11] Even with proper injection technique, patients may experience a dropped lip, decrease pursing of the lips, a change in speech, or oral incompetence.[11] Chin hyperhidrosis is treated effectively with 2 units per injection.[11] Patients can have oral incompetence, dropped chin, or an asymmetric smile. The typical doses of BoNT-A required per facial locale are summarized in **Table 2**. Overall, side effects are uncommon with good injection technique and when small doses are used. Side effects are typically minimal, and depend on the area of injection (**Table 3**).[2,14] The duration of benefit may be shorter when treating facial hyperhidrosis and patients should plan on treatments 2 to 3 times per year.

FREY SYNDROME (GUSTATORY SWEATING)

Frey syndrome, known as gustatory sweating, presents with sweating and/or flushing of the preauricular and mandibular areas from injury to the parotid gland. Parotid injury is most commonly unilateral, and is seen after surgical procedures such as parotidectomy and face lift surgery, or less commonly from neuropathy associated with diabetes. In a recent population-based study, 3% of patients after parotidectomy developed Frey syndrome that required treatment after a mean of 9.6 months.[15] Frey syndrome is thought to be caused by aberrant regeneration of the parasympathetic nerves innervating the sweat glands.[16,17] The abnormal sweating on the face can appear when the person eats, sees, or even thinks about certain foods that produce strong salivation. Frey syndrome has been well studied, and there is consensus regarding the safety and efficacy of BoNT-A therapy.[16]

Eliciting a history of gustatory sweating in a patient several months after parotidectomy, or surgical face lift, is sufficient to diagnose most patients. A starch-iodine test can be performed to confirm the problem (**Fig. 4**) and to identify the area of involvement.[16] After the skin is prepped with iodine and corn starch powder, the patient can be asked to eat food known to provoke sweating in that patient, such as sweet or tart foods, or chewing gum.[17]

Compared with the other areas of facial sweating, there is more substantial literature supporting the efficacy of both abo-BoNT-A and ona-BoNT-A. Abo-BoNT-A, at 10 to 20 units per 1 cm^2 of affected skin, can effectively reduce gustatory sweating for 8 to 16.5 months.[16,18] Likewise, 1.5 units of ona-BoNT-A per 1 cm^2, for a total average dose of 38 units, can effectively reduce gustatory sweating for an average of 15 months.[17] However, there is great variability in the duration of effectiveness reported in the literature, and it seems to be independent of age, sex, or extent of parotidectomy.[16,17] In our experience, it is common for patients to achieve remission for 1 to 3 years and doses can range from 15 to 100 units of ona-BoNT-A. The affected area is treated with 2.5 to 3 units injected every 1 to 1.5 cm. There are few side effects with BoNT-A treatment. Dry mouth and a potential to cause temporary weakness with mastication have been reported.[17] Smile asymmetry is also possible.

SUBMAMMARY HYPERHIDROSIS

There is a lack of published data regarding the prevalence and treatment of submammary hyperhidrosis. Patients frequently have difficulty pinpointing the area of sweating because the sweat solution spreads along the chest wall, and even down to the abdomen. Starch-iodine testing is helpful for localizing the affected areas for treatment. In our experience, ona-BoNT-A at 2.5 units per injection, spaced evenly at 1.5 to 2 cm per injection, is effective for this region. There are times when a positive starch-iodine test cannot be elicited, in which case we treat an area 2 to 4 cm inferior and superior to the submammary crease, from the midline of the inferior chest/upper abdomen to the lateral edge of the breast or sometimes to the

Table 2 Craniofacial hyperhidrosis: typical doses of ona-BoNT-A				
Facial Area	Units Per Injection	Spacing of Injections (cm)	Average Total Dose (units)	Average Duration of Effectiveness (mo)
Forehead and anterior scalp	2–3	2	100	4–6
Ophiasis scalp	2.5	2	100	4–6
Scalp and forehead	2–2.5	2	300	4–6
Nose	1–2	0.5–1	10–20	3–6
Upper lip	2	0.5–1	10	3–6
Chin	2	0.5–1	10	3–6

Table 3
Side effects of botulinum toxin injection of the face/scalp

Common Adverse Events	Uncommon Adverse Events
Injection site pain	Brow or eyelid ptosis
Bruising/erythema	Malaise
Swelling	Ectropion
Headache	Xerophthalmia
Local paresthesia	Blepharoptosis
Asymmetry	Oral incompetence
	Diplopia

Data from Glaser DA, Hebert AA, Pariser DM, et al. Facial hyperhidrosis: best practice recommendations and special considerations. Cutis 2007;79(Suppl 5):29–32; and Dorizas A, Krueger N, Sadick NS. Aesthetic uses of the botulinum toxin. Dermatol Clin 2014;32(1):23–36.

midaxillary line. Because of the variations in size of the thorax and submammary region, a total of 50 to 150 units of ona-BoNT-A may be required per affected side.

HYPERHIDROSIS OF THE GROIN

There are few published reports regarding hyperhidrosis of the groin. The inguinal folds, perineum, gluteal cleft, anal fold, and buttocks can be affected. Patients complain of and present with sweating in the groin area. Patients may complain of wet underwear and clothing, as well as leaving wet marks on surfaces after sitting. Patients can have noticeably wet areas on their clothes at presentation. The starch-iodine test helps to localize the area of sweating in these locations, but can be challenging to perform in areas such as the

gluteal cleft/anal fold.[19] An example of a positive starch-iodine test of the inguinal fold, and marking the area for injection, is given in **Fig. 5**. A positive starch-iodine test of the anal fold is shown in **Fig. 6**.

The ideal dose of botulinum toxin for these regions has not been established. Several case reports have found that 2 to 3 units of ona-BoNT-A injected 1 to 2 cm apart, for a total of 50 units per inguinal fold, is effective for inguinal hyperhidrosis.[20–22] If a starch-iodine test is negative, we inject ~2 cm medial and 2 cm lateral to the inguinal crease, making sure to avoid injection of the labia minor. The effects of treatment typically last 3 to 6 months.[20,21] The few reported side effects are related to the injections, and include temporary edema and small hematoma formation.[20]

A prospective trial of 11 patients[19] showed effective ona-BoNT-A treatment of anal fold hyperhidrosis. One unit of ona-BoNT-A was injected at 1-cm intervals, for a total dose range of 30 to 54 units, depending on the size of the involved area. With the exception of pain with injections, no other side effects of treatment were noted, even with the proximity to the anal sphincter. When injecting this area, the authors try to stay 1 to 2 cm lateral to the anal verge to prevent diffusion of BoNT-A into the anal sphincter. We have not seen anal incompetence after injecting the gluteal cleft/anal fold, although it is important to review the possible risk of temporary fecal incontinence with each patient.

HYPERHIDROSIS OF AMPUTATED LIMBS

Hyperhidrosis is reported in 23% to 56% of limb amputees, and has a significant impact on their

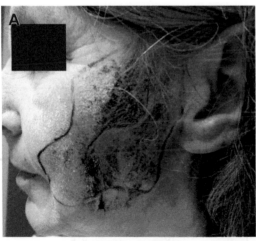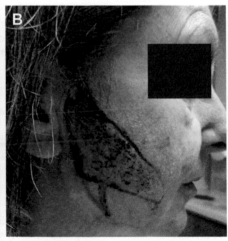

Fig. 4. A patient with bilateral Frey syndrome showing the variation in the affected surface area on each side (*A* and *B*), which highlights the importance of performing a starch-iodine test.

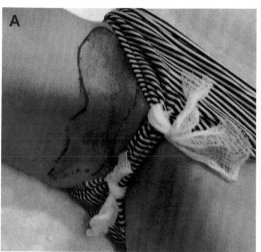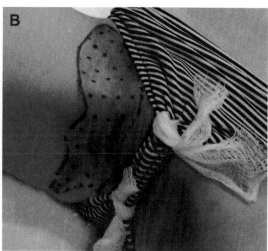

Fig. 5. A positive starch-iodine test of the inguinal fold (*A*), and an example of how to properly mark the inguinal fold for botulinum toxin injection (*B*). (*Courtesy of* Albert Ganss, International Hyperhidrosis Society, Quakertown, PA; with permission.)

quality of life.[23] The excess sweating can interfere with the prosthesis fitting comfortably and properly. The exact pathophysiology is unknown, and is likely multifactorial. It is possible that the remaining sweat glands in the surgical area compensate for the decreased amount of secretory tissue.[24] The use of nonpermeable suction stockings and silicone liners within the prosthesis exacerbates the problem.[23,25]

Patients report that perspiration depends on friction and physical exertion, rather than temperature.[23,26] A starch-iodine test pinpoints the areas of excess sweating, and allows more precise treatment. In this patient cohort, the iodine and starch are applied as usual, but the patient may need to apply the prosthesis for several minutes in order to produce the most accurate results.[26]

Ona-BoNT-A, at 2 to 3 units per injection, is injected circumferentially at 1-cm to 2-cm intervals within the identified area of the amputee's socket.[25,26] The total amount of ona-BoNT-A varies depending on the affected limb, but can be as high as 300 to 500 units per treatment.[25] Treatment effectiveness and duration vary, but can last from 4 to 12 months.[26,27] Kern and colleagues[23] found that a total of 1750 units of botulinum neurotoxin-B (BoNT-B), injected into 20 spots, spaced at 2-cm to 4-cm intervals, was effective at controlling limb hyperhidrosis for 3 months (end of study visit).[23] The investigators concluded that BoNT-B seems to be as effective as BoNT-A but has a wider area of diffusion, which may be beneficial for the large areas involved in amputated limbs.

Because low doses of BoNT-B are required for treatment of hyperhidrosis, in contrast with doses of 5000 units or greater for cervical dystonia, the autonomic side effects were few and minimal.[23] Reported autonomic side effects of BoNT-B included dry mouth, blurry vision, and dry nasal mucosa.[23] Side effects of ona-BoNT-A treatment are minimal, and include small hematomas at the sites of injection and injection pain.[26] A botulinum toxin type A is preferred by the authors to minimize the risks of systemic side effects.

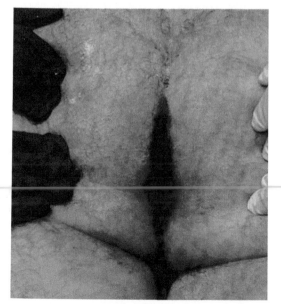

Fig. 6. A positive starch-iodine test of the anal fold.

COMPENSATORY HYPERHIDROSIS

Compensatory hyperhidrosis (CHH) is seen in 60% to 90% of patients after treatment of severe axillary and/or palmar HH with thoracic sympathectomy.[28,29] Approximately 40% of patients have CHH, for which treatment is sought.[28] The mechanism for CHH is unclear, and there is no accurate way to predict which patient may have this entity after sympathectomy. CHH most commonly affects the back (**Fig. 7**), abdomen, and chest, but the groin and thighs are common areas as well. CHH can be more debilitating and intolerable than the primary hyperhidrosis, and it is thought to be irreversible.[30] CHH may be irreversible, even in cases after surgical clip removal, which has been seen in 2 prospective clinical trials.[24,31]

The patient can help identify the most troubling regions of CHH, and a starch-iodine test should be used to define the size of the areas to be treated. Ona-BoNT-A is an effective therapy that can last an average of 4 months per treatment.[30] Patient outcomes tend to be less satisfying for CHH than for other body areas already discussed, probably from under dosing because the surface areas tend to be so large. Injections are spaced 1 to 2 cm apart using 2.5 units per injection site. The total amount of ona-BoNT-A can vary from 100 to 500 units, depending on the surface area involved.[30,32] Doses of ona-BoNT-A are generally limited to 300 to 400 units per session to minimize the risk of side effects. Concurrent therapy with topical antiperspirants and/or oral anticholinergics may be necessary. Minor injection site pain is the most common side effect.

SUMMARY

Botulinum toxin-A therapy is an effective treatment option for patients with primary or secondary focal hyperhidrosis. The amount of BoNT-A required per treatment, and the duration of effectiveness, vary with the area of hyperhidrosis. Accurate identification of the area of excess sweating with a starch-iodine test can help maximize outcomes. Injections placed at the dermal-subcutaneous junction ensure the best efficacy, minimize muscular uptake, and reduce the risks of local muscle weakness. Repeat treatments are necessary and botulinum toxin injections can be combined with other hyperhidrosis therapy.

REFERENCES

1. Lear W, Kessler E, Solish N, et al. An epidemiological study of hyperhidrosis. Dermatol Surg 2007; 33(s1):S69–75.
2. Glaser DA, Hebert AA, Pariser DM, et al. Facial hyperhidrosis: best practice recommendations and special considerations. Cutis 2007;79(Suppl 5): 29–32.
3. Rystedt A, Swartling C, Naver H. Anhidrotic effect of intradermal injections of botulinum toxin: a comparison of different products and concentrations. Acta Derm Venereol 2008;88(3):229–33.
4. El Kahky HM, Diab HM, Aly DG, et al. Efficacy of onabotulinum toxin A (Botox) versus abobotulinum toxin A (Dysport) using a conversion factor (1: 2.5) in treatment of primary palmar hyperhidrosis. Dermatol Res Pract 2013;2013:1–6.
5. Vergilis-Kalner IJ. Same-patient prospective comparison of Botox versus Dysport for the treatment of primary axillary hyperhidrosis and review of literature. J Drugs Dermatol 2011;10(9):1013–5.
6. Rosell K, Hymnelius K, Swartling C. Botulinum toxin type A and B improve quality of life in patients with axillary and palmar hyperhidrosis. Acta Derm Venereol 2013;93(3):335–9.
7. Campanati A, Giuliodori K, Giuliano A, et al. Treatment of palmar hyperhidrosis with botulinum toxin type A: results of a pilot study based on a novel injective approach. Arch Dermatol Res 2013; 305(8):691–7.

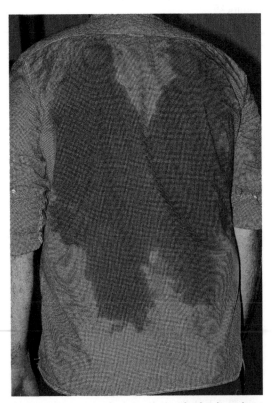

Fig. 7. CHH commonly presents on the back and can affect a large surface area, making treatment challenging.

8. Hsu TS, Dover JS, Arndt KA. Effect of volume and concentration on the diffusion of botulinum exotoxin A. Arch Dermatol 2004;140(11):1351–4.

9. Trindade De Almeida AR, Marques E, De Almeida J, et al. Pilot study comparing the diffusion of two formulations of botulinum toxin type A in patients with forehead hyperhidrosis. Dermatol Surg 2007; 33(s1):S37–43.

10. Anders D, Moosbauer S, Naumann MK, et al. Craniofacial hyperhidrosis successfully treated with botulinum toxin type A. Eur J Dermatol 2008;18(1): 87–8.

11. George SM, Atkinson LR, Farrant PB, et al. Botulinum toxin for focal hyperhidrosis of the face. Br J Dermatol 2014;170(1):211–3. Available at: http://onlinelibrary. wiley.com/doi/10.1111/bjd.12568/abstract. Accessed November 19, 2013.

12. Geddoa E, Balakumar AK, Paes TR. The successful use of botulinum toxin for the treatment of nasal hyperhidrosis. Int J Dermatol 2008;47(10):1079–80.

13. Komericki P, Ardjomand N. Hyperhidrosis of face and scalp: repeated successful treatment with botulinum toxin type A. Indian J Dermatol Venereol Leprol 2012;78(2):201.

14. Dorizas A, Krueger N, Sadick NS. Aesthetic uses of the botulinum toxin. Dermatol Clin 2014;32(1):23–36.

15. Moeller K, Esser D, Boeger D, et al. Parotidectomy and submandibulectomy for benign diseases in Thuringia, Germany: a population-based study on epidemiology and outcome. Eur Arch Oto Rhino Laryngol 2012;270(3):1149–55.

16. Steffen A, Rotter N, König IR, et al. Botulinum toxin for Frey's syndrome: a closer look at different treatment responses. J Laryngol Otol 2011;126(2):185–9.

17. Díaz PM, del Castillo RB, de la Plata MM, et al. Clinical results in the management of Frey's Syndrome with injections of botulinum toxin. Med Oral Patol Oral Cir Bucal 2008;13:E248–52.

18. Guntinas-Lichius O. Increased botulinum toxin type A dosage is more effective in patients with Frey's syndrome. Laryngoscope 2002;112(4):746–9.

19. Bechara FG, Sand M, Achenbach RK, et al. Focal hyperhidrosis of the anal fold: successful treatment with botulinum toxin A. Dermatol Surg 2007;33(8): 924–7.

20. Hexsel DM, Dal'forno T, Hexsel CL. Inguinal, or Hexsel's hyperhidrosis. Clin Dermatol 2004;22(1):53–9.

21. Woolery-Lloyd H, Elsaie ML, Avashia N. Inguinal hyperhidrosis misdiagnosed as urinary incontinence: treatment with botulinum toxin A. J Drugs Dermatol 2008;7(3):293–5.

22. Barankin B, Wasel N. Treatment of inguinal hyperhidrosis with botulinum toxin type A. Int J Dermatol 2006;45(8):985–6.

23. Kern U, Kohl M, Seifert U, et al. Botulinum toxin type B in the treatment of residual limb hyperhidrosis for lower limb amputees: a pilot study. Am J P M R 2011;90(4):321–9.

24. Sugimura H, Spratt EH, Compeau CG, et al. Thoracoscopic sympathetic clipping for hyperhidrosis: long-term results and reversibility. J Thorac Cardiovasc Surg 2009;137(6):1370–8.

25. Charrow A, DiFazio M, Foster L, et al. Intradermal botulinum toxin type A injection effectively reduces residual limb hyperhidrosis in amputees: a case series. Arch Phys Med Rehabil 2008;89(7):1407–9.

26. Gratrix M, Hivnor C. Botulinum toxin A treatment for hyperhidrosis in patients with prosthetic limbs. Arch Dermatol 2010;146(11):1314.

27. García-Morales I, Pérez-Bernal A, Camacho F. Letter: stump hyperhidrosis in a leg amputee: treatment with botulinum toxin A. Dermatol Surg 2007;33(11): 1401–2.

28. Currie AC, Evans JR, Thomas PR. An analysis of the natural course of compensatory sweating following thoracoscopic sympathectomy. Int J Surg 2011; 9(5):437–9.

29. Deng B, Tan QY, Jiang YG, et al. Optimization of sympathectomy to treat palmar hyperhidrosis: the systematic review and meta-analysis of studies published during the past decade. Surg Endosc 2010; 25(6):1893–901.

30. Kim WO, Kil HK, Yoon KB, et al. Botulinum toxin: a treatment for compensatory hyperhidrosis in the trunk. Dermatol Surg 2009;35(5):833–8.

31. Findikcioglu A, Kilic D, Hatipoglu A. Is clipping superior to cauterization in the treatment of palmar hyperhidrosis? Thorac Cardiovasc Surg 2013. [Epub ahead of print].

32. Santana-Rodríguez N, Clavo B, Calatayud-Gastardi J, et al. Severe compensatory hyperhidrosis following thoracic sympathectomy successfully treated with low doses of botulinum toxin A. J Dermatolog Treat 2012;23(6):457–60.

Oral Medications

Dee Anna Glaser, MD

KEYWORDS

- Systemic therapy • Anticholinergic • β-blocker • Glycopyrrolate • Oxybutynin • Propanolol
- Clonidine • Hyperhidrosis

KEY POINTS

- Localized treatments for hyperhidrosis are considered first-line therapy.
- Systemic therapy can be used as monotherapy or in combination with focally targeted treatments.
- Anticholinergic drugs are the most commonly used systemic therapy for hyperhidrosis.
- Side effect profiles of anticholinergic drugs vary based on their lipid solubility.
- β-Blockers can be useful for hyperhidrosis associated with performance tasks.
- There is a paucity of published literature on systemic treatment of hyperhidrosis.

INTRODUCTION

Hyperhidrosis (HH) is a disabling condition that impacts quality of life (QOL) and can cause significant emotional stress. Primary HH presents with focal areas of excess sweating, such as the axillae, palms, soles, scalp, face, and groin. Although some patients have only one focal area of excessive sweating, it is common for patients to have more than one body site producing excessive amounts of sweat.[1] In addition, patients may present with more generalized forms of HH, which are usually secondary in nature. In these cases, treatment or removal of the offending cause is beneficial, but may not always be feasible. Compensatory HH following sympathectomy varies significantly but occurs in 50% to 80% of patients who undergo sympathectomy.[2] It can affect very large areas, such as the chest, abdomen, and back, and is irreversible. Systemic therapy can be beneficial in all of these patients.

None of these agents have a Food and Drug Administration–approved indication to treat HH and there is a paucity of literature or studies on the use of these medications for the treatment of HH.

TREATMENT INDICATIONS

In general, treatment of primary HH should be as specific and focal or localized as possible to ensure good response and minimize side effects and interactions with other medications. Topical therapies are usually first-line treatment, and then more focally targeted therapies, such as botulinum toxin injections, iontophoresis, or microwave thermolysis, should be considered. However, when these treatments are ineffective, intolerable, or not feasible, systemic therapies are a good option. Oral medications can be added to the previously mentioned treatments to enhance improvements. This is especially beneficial when patients have multiple areas of HH. I might use botulinum toxin A injections for the axilla and iontophoresis for the hands and feet, but have to add an oral agent to manage such areas as the groin, face, or submammary sweating.

Generalized sweating presents a challenge. If a specific cause is identified, that agent or cause should be removed. However, it is common that an offending agent cannot be removed. Patients with psychiatric disease frequently cannot lower or change the medications that are controlling their

Disclosure: D.A. Glaser has served as advisor for Allergan, Galderma, Miramar Labs, and Unilever. She has been an investigator and received research grants from Allergan, Miramar Labs, and Ulthera.
Department of Dermatology, Saint Louis University School of Medicine, 1402 South Grand Boulevard-ABI, St Louis, MO 63104, USA
E-mail address: glasermd@slu.edu

Dermatol Clin 32 (2014) 527–532
http://dx.doi.org/10.1016/j.det.2014.06.002
0733-8635/14/$ – see front matter

derm.theclinics.com

mental illness. In these instances, other options, such as oral medications to treat the HH, have to be considered.[3] Some patients have multiple cofounding factors that can induce or worsen HH, and in these patients oral therapy may be very helpful.

There are groups of patients that should be considered very carefully before initiating therapy with oral medications, especially the oral anticholinergics, which decrease sweating from the entire body. Athletes and individuals who work or play a lot outdoors may become overheated if they are unable to cool their bodies without sweat evaporation, and may have an increased risk of hyperthermia and heat stroke. Small children or individuals who have difficulty self-monitoring their body temperature, mentation, and urine output may not be good candidates for oral anticholinergics. Allergies, other medications, or health issues need to be reviewed to avoid interactions or worsening of other diseases or health concerns. As an example, β-blockers are generally not given to patients with psoriasis.

It is very important to counsel patients on what therapy you are using, how it works, and what to monitor. It is also critical that patients are counseled on realistic expectations. Most patients can expect an improvement but not complete resolution of their HH symptoms. I counsel patients that they will most likely still have episodes of sweating when others around them do not, and that they will most likely still be the first to sweat and even sweat more than their counterparts during activity. Setting a step-wise plan for the patient can also be helpful so that they do not discontinue therapy and understand that if a plan is not providing enough improvement, then the next step will be added, especially with oral therapies. Improvement in symptoms is usually possible to achieve, but anhidrosis is not, nor is it desirable.

ANTICHOLINERGIC AGENTS

Because the sweat glands are innervated by the sympathetic postganglionic nerves and have acetylcholine as the primary neurotransmitter, the use of anticholinergic agents is a logical choice to treat HH.[4] Anticholinergic agents work by competitive inhibition of acetylcholine at the muscarinic receptor. Muscarinic receptors are present throughout the central and autonomic nervous system, accounting for widespread and varied side effects that can develop.

There are several anticholinergic agents; however, there are differences in the side effect profile. Glycopyrrolate is a quaternary amine with limited passage across lipid membranes, such as the blood-brain barrier. This is in contrast to such agents as atropine or scopolamine, which are tertiary amines and can easily penetrate lipid barriers. This is probably the reason why glycopyrrolate has fewer central nervous system side effects and may have less effect on the heart rate at lower doses.[5] The most common side effect is dry mouth caused by inhibition of salivary glands. There are many potential side effects (**Box 1**) and concurrent use with other medications with anticholinergic activity, such as phenothiazines, antiparkinson drugs, or tricyclic antidepressants, intensifies the antimuscarinic effects and increases side effects. Anticholinergic therapy may be contraindicated in patients with glaucoma, obstructive uropathy, obstructive diseases of the gastrointestinal (GI) tract, paralytic ileus, severe ulcerative colitis, and myasthenia gravis.

Glycopyrrolate

Glycopyrrolate is the author's most commonly used anticholinergic drug to treat HH. Dosing is variable and is usually started at 1 to 2 mg twice daily (BID). The patient is asked to increase the dose by 1 mg per day at 2-week intervals based on the therapeutic response and side effects. Dry mouth is the most common side effect and usually the limiting factor in dosing. If side effects are minimal, management can allow patients to continue their medication. Managing dry mouth could include use of artificial saliva preparations, increasing water intake, and keeping candy or mints available; increased fiber consumption and light exercise can help to improve mild constipation. Over-the-counter eye drops can improve dry eye symptoms, but many patients have to discontinue therapy because of intolerable side effects. The efficacy and side effects of therapy are generally dose-dependent.

Walling[6] published a retrospective review of 45 patients who used glycopyrrolate to treat HH of various body sites. Overall 67% were responders and 33% failed treatment. Of the treatment failures, 40% were nonresponders and the rest had adverse effects requiring medication cessation (xerostomia, GI disturbance, headache, rash, and mental status change). Only one-fourth of his patients used it as monotherapy, but others combined therapy with topical aluminum chloride, botulinum toxin, and iontophoresis. His patients most commonly took 1 mg daily and the highest dose that was used was 6 mg daily. Bajaj and Langtry[5] reported on 19 patients treated with glycopyrrolate and found that 80% responded to therapy. The most common dose was 2 mg BID or three times daily (TID) but one patient took

Box 1
Anticholinergic therapy side effects

Gastrointestinal

Dry mouth

Constipation

Nausea

Vomiting

Bloated feeling

Loss of taste

Ocular

Mydriasis

Cycloplegia

Dry or gritty eyes

Blurred vision

Photophobia

Respiratory

Bronchodilation

Reduced secretions

Genitourinary

Urinary retention

Slow voiding

Urinary hesitancy

Erectile dysfunction

Loss of libido

Cardiac

Bradycardia (lower doses)

Tachycardia (higher doses)

Arrhythmias

Palpitations

Central nervous system

Headache

Dizziness

Insomnia

Drowsiness

Mental confusion and/or excitement (usually in elderly)

Seizures

Skin

Decreased sweating

Urticaria

Pruritus

4 mg BID. Side effects were reported in 80% of the patients and about one-third of their patients had to stop the glycopyrrolate because of side effects. Typically my patients require daily maintenance, but a few take it on an "as-needed basis." Doses range from 1 to 8 mg BID and do not seem to correlate significantly with age, gender, or body mass.

Oxybutynin

Oxybutynin is another common anticholinergic drug that is used to treat HH. It is classified as a tertiary amine. It comes in several different preparations including a tablet, slow-release tablet, topical gel, and transdermal patch. For oral administration, 5 to 10 mg daily is usually required for relief of HH, but doses up to 15 or 20 mg daily may be required.[7,8] Wolosker and coworkers[9] did a randomized placebo-controlled trial using oxybutynin for palmar and axillary HH. Fifty patients were enrolled, and the drug was initiated at 2.5 mg daily, increased to 2.5 mg BID during weeks 2 and 3, and then treated with 5 mg BID. Approximately 70% of the patients reported improvement in their axillary and palmar HH, whereas 90% of patients with plantar involvement reported improvement in their plantar sweating. Most of the treated patients reported improvement in their QOL, whereas one-fourth had no change in their QOL. Side effects were limited to dry mouth that was rated as moderate to severe by 30% of the subjects during the first 3 weeks (lower dose) and reached 35% by 6 weeks with the higher dose of oxybutynin. Tupker and coworkers[8] reported 13 patients with generalized HH and 1 with drug-induced HH that were treated with oxybutynin (2.5 mg TID, and 5 mg TID), with all of the generalized HH patients responding (the paroxetine-induced HH patient did not respond). Therapy was well tolerated with the most common side effects being dry mouth, urinary difficulty, GI complaints, headache, and lassitude, although 30% had to discontinue therapy because of side effects. Therapy seems to work well in men and women, and overweight and obese individuals.[10,11]

There are no guidelines to use when choosing which anticholinergic drug to use for HH. Because of the more limited penetration into the central nervous system, glycopyrrolate is a good option. Patients may respond to one anticholinergic drug better than another, or may experience fewer or different side effects with one drug compared with other anticholinergics.[6] Additionally, there may be better compliance with the once-daily slow-release oxybutynin. It is reasonable to switch anticholinergic drugs when faced with non-response. Another option is to try a topical formulation.

Other Anticholinergic Agents

Other drugs with antimuscarinic effects can be used to treat HH, and different options are available in various parts of the world. One of the best studied is methantheline bromide, which is a quaternary amine available in Germany. A large multicenter placebo-controlled randomized study of 339 patients with axillary or palmar-axillary HH was performed.[12] Methantheline, 50 mg, or placebo was used TID and gravimetric measurements of sweat, Hyperhidrosis Disease Severity Scale, and QOL were measured. At Day 28, there was a reduction of sweat production of 40% compared with the placebo, although the measured reduction in sweat production was greater in the axilla as compared with the palms. The researchers hypothesized that the decreased efficacy in the palmar sweating may be because a significant proportion of methantheline is excreted through the sebaceous glands and these are lacking in the palms. There was good tolerability with dry mouth, impaired accommodation, and dry eyes reported. There was a statistically significant decrease in the Hyperhidrosis Disease Severity Scale and an improvement in QOL in methantheline-treated subjects.

Anticholinergic Use in Pediatric Patients

In general, I avoid the use of systemic anticholinergic therapy for my young patients with HH because they have less control of their environment at school, may be exposed to heat stresses during playtime, and may not be able to monitor themselves for signs or symptoms of hyperthermia. However, Paller and coworkers[13] reported on 31 pediatric patients that were treated with glycopyrrolate and found that 90% had improvement and 10% had no improvement in their HH. The average age of her patients at the time that the glycopyrrolate was prescribed was 14.8 years ± 2.9. The mean dose for these teenagers was 2 mg daily but ranged from 1 to 6 mg daily. Approximately 30% had side effects including dry mouth, dry eyes, and blurred vision. One patient had to stop therapy because of palpitations. Oxybutynin has been studied extensively in children for urologic problems with a good safety profile, although there is a higher number of central nervous system adverse event cases reported in pediatric patients as compared with adult patients.[14,15] Glycopyrrolate is approved by the Food and Drug Administration to treat children with sialorrhea and in this

population side effects are dose-dependent and include behavioral changes, constipation, excessively dry mouth, urinary retention, facial flushing, nasal congestion, vomiting, and diarrhea.[16]

β-ADRENERGIC BLOCKERS

The use of β-blockers to treat patients with HH stems from their use to improve symptoms of social phobias and performance anxiety.[17] Episodes of HH may develop throughout the day, but many patients complain that the sweating develops at times of performance-related stress or just a perception that sweating may interfere with performance, such as meetings, public speaking, or school performance. In these instances the use of a β-blocker, such as propranolol, can be helpful. Propranolol is a highly lipophilic drug that binds to β1 and β2 receptors with equal affinity. Peak concentration is 1 to 1.5 hours postingestion, although food may delay peak concentration.[18] Contraindications to therapy are numerous (**Box 2**) and a thorough history needs to be obtained, but low doses are generally used infrequently, making this therapy well tolerated. A resting blood pressure and heart rate should be taken in the office before prescribing the drug.

Commonly used doses are 10 to 20 mg of propranolol taken approximately 1 hour before the

---

Box 2
Contraindications for propranolol

Bradycardia[a]

AV block[a]

Asthma

Chronic obstructive pulmonary disease

Depression

Diabetes mellitus

Heart failure

Hepatic disease

Hypotension

Hypoglycemia

Cerebrovascular disease

Myasthenia gravis

Psoriasis

Renal disease

Thyroid disease

Elderly

Driving or operating machinery

[a] Absolute contraindication.

planned performance. For patients with low resting blood pressure, slow baseline heart rates, or very small body mass index, 5 mg may be used initially. Patients should take a "test run" at home to monitor for hypotension, orthostatic hypotension, depressed cognition, or poor performance in general.

α-ADRENERGIC AGONIST

Clonidine is a sympatholytic medication used to treat hypertension and some anxiety/panic disorders. It is classified as a centrally acting α_2-adrenergic agonist and has been successfully used to treat some patients with HH, and with flushing and sweating associated with menopause.[6,19–21] Doses used to treat menopausal hot flashes were low, ranging from 0.025 to 0.1 mg BID. Walling's[6] reported dose in 13 patients with HH was 0.1 mg BID. Overall there was a 46% response rate and most of his patients used clonidine as monotherapy. Interestingly, the patients with craniofacial HH comprised most of his responders. Of the seven patients who failed treatment, three were nonresponders and four had to discontinue the medication because of side effects related to decreased blood pressure. Side effects most commonly seen with the use of clonidine are dry mouth, dizziness, constipation, and sedation.

As with propranolol, a thorough history and examination including blood pressure should be performed before initiating therapy. Doses of 0.1 mg BID are most commonly used and the drug can be combined with other therapies to treat HH.[6,21] Anecdotally, I have found it most useful in my middle-aged patients with craniofacial HH and sweating associated with flushing. I have prescribed it for generalized HH especially when there are several factors contributing to the overall sweating.

BENZODIAZEPINES

Benzodiazepines are sometimes listed as a treatment of HH, social anxiety disorders, and performance anxiety.[17,22] Diazepam, 5 to 20 mg/day, is recommended, but there is no real primary literature supporting the efficacy in patients with HH. Because HH is a chronic disease, one has to carefully weigh the risks of addiction or dependence. Propanolol is the author's first choice to treat performance-based sweating. If anxiety seems to be the overriding problem, referral to psychiatry for cognitive therapy or other drug management is prudent.

OTHER SYSTEMIC AGENTS

There are a few anecdotal case reports using other systemic agents to help reduce sweating of various etiologies, which may be of use in limited situations, or when other therapies have not produced satisfactory improvement.

The calcium channel blocker, diltiazem, was been reported to improve palmar sweating in two family members with autosomal-dominant emotional HH.[23] A woman with "lifelong generalized HH" reported resolution of sweating when treated with indomethacin, 25 mg TID, for her arthritis.[24] Gabapentin when used with probantheline improved sweating in a child suffering from HH after a spinal cord injury.[25] Gabapentin has also been used with limited success in social anxiety disorder.[17]

SUMMARY

Oral therapies can play an important role in treating HH of all types. Although monotherapy is sometimes useful, combining systemic treatments with more focally based therapy may provide superior results. Because of side effects and drug interactions, a thorough assessment should be performed before initiating systemic therapy, and working with other health care team members is valuable to monitor for and reduce the risks of systemic therapies.

REFERENCES

1. Lear W, Kessler E, Solish N, et al. An epidemiological study of hyperhidrosis. Dermatol Surg 2007; 33(1 Spec No):S69–75.
2. Cerfolio RJ, De Campos JR, Bryant AS, et al. The Society of Thoracic Surgeons expert consensus for the surgical treatment of hyperhidrosis. Ann Thorac Surg 2011;91(5):1642–8.
3. Mago R. Glycopyrrolate for antidepressant-associated excessive sweating. J Clin Psychopharmacol 2013;33(2):279–80.
4. Lakraj AD, Moghimi N, Jabbari B. Hyperhidrosis: anatomy, pathophysiology and treatment with emphasis on the role of botulinum toxins. Toxins (Basel) 2013;5:821–40.
5. Bajaj V, Langtry JA. Use of oral glycopyrronium bromide in hyperhidrosis. Br J Dermatol 2007; 157:118–21.
6. Walling HW. Systemic therapy for primary hyperhidrosis: a retrospective study of 59 patients treated with glycopyrrolate or clonidine. J Am Acad Dermatol 2012;66(3):387–92.
7. Messikh R, Elkhyat A, Aubin F, et al. Use of oral oxybutynin at 7.5 mg per day in primary hyperhidrosis. Rev Med Liege 2012;67(10):520–6 [in French].
8. Tupker RA, Harmsze AM, Deneer VHM. Oxybutynin therapy for generalized hyperhidrosis. Arch Dermatol 2006;148(8):1065–86.

9. Wolokser N, de Campos JR, Kauffman P, et al. A randomized placebo-controlled trial of oxybutynin for the initial treatment of palmar and axillary hyperhidrosis. J Vasc Surg 2012;55(6):1696–700.

10. Wolosker N, Krutman M, Campdell TP, et al. Oxybutynin treatment for hyperhidrosis: a comparative analysis between genders. Einstein (Sao Paulo) 2012;10(4):405–8.

11. Wolosker N, Krutman M, Kauffman P, et al. Oxybutynin treatment for hyperhidrosis in overweight and obese patients. Rev Assoc Med Bras 2013; 59(2):143–7.

12. Müller C, Berensmeier A, Hamm H, et al. Efficacy and safety of methantheline bromide (vagantin) in axillary and palmar hyperhidrosis: results from a multicenter, randomized, placebo-controlled trial. J Eur Acad Dermatol Venereol 2013;27:1278–84.

13. Paller AS, Shah PR, Silverio AM, et al. Oral glycopyrrolate as second-line treatment for primary pediatric hyperhidrosis. J Am Acad Dermatol 2012;67(5): 918–23.

14. Armstrong RB, Dmochowski RR, Sand PK, et al. Safety and tolerability of extended-release oxybutynin once daily in urinary incontinence: combined results from two phase 4 controlled clinical trials. Int Urol Nephrol 2007;39(4):1069–77.

15. Gish P, Mosholder AD, Truffa M, et al. Spectrum of central anticholinergic adverse effects associated with oxybutynin: comparison of pediatric and adult cases. J Pediatr 2009;155(3):432–4.

16. Mier RJ, Bachrach SJ, Lakin RC, et al. Treatment of sialorrhea with glycopyrrolate: a double-blind dose-ranging study. Arch Pediatr Adolesc Med 2000; 154(12):1214–8.

17. Schneier RF. Social anxiety disorder. N Engl J Med 2006;355:1029–36.

18. Brown J, Laiken N. Chapter 9, Muscarinic receptor agonists and antagonists. In: Brunton LL, Chabner BA, Knollmann BC, editors. Goodman & Gilman's the pharmacological basis of therapeutics. 12th edition. New York, NY: McGraw-Hill; 2011. Available at: http://accessmedicine.mhmedical.com.ezp.slu.edu/content.aspx?bookid=374&Sectionid=41266215. Accessed July 24, 2014.

19. Feder R. Clonidine treatment of excessive sweating. J Clin Psychiatry 1995;56(1):35.

20. Nelson HD, Vesco KK, Haney E, et al. Nonhormonal therapies for menopausal hot flashes: systematic review and meta-analysis. JAMA 2006; 295(17):2057–71.

21. Torch EM. Remission of facial and scalp hyperhidrosis with clonidine hydrochloride and topical aluminum chloride. South Med J 2000;93(1):68–9.

22. Böni R. Generalized hyperhidrosis and its systemic treatment. Curr Probl Dermatol 2002;30:44–7.

23. James WD, Schoomaker EB, Rodman OC. Emotional eccrine sweating. A heritable disorder. Arch Dermatol 1987;123(7):925–9.

24. Tkach JR. Indomethacin treatment of generalized hyperhidrosis. J Am Acad Dermatol 1982;6(4):545.

25. Adams BB, Vargus-Adams JN, Franz DN, et al. Hyperhidrosis in pediatric spinal cord injury: a case report and gabapentin therapy. J Am Acad Dermatol 2002;46(3):444–6.

Local Procedural Approaches for Axillary Hyperhidrosis

Dee Anna Glaser, MD*, Timur A. Galperin, DO

KEYWORDS

- Hyperhidrosis • Liposuction-curettage • Microwave thermolysis • Minimally invasive • Surgery

KEY POINTS

- Surgical procedures can provide long-lasting relief from axillary hyperhidrosis.
- Local or tumescent anesthesia is most commonly used for local procedures of the axilla.
- Most of these procedures are limited to treating the axillary region of the body.
- Starch-iodine testing is valuable to identify the area of treatment, but the hair-bearing skin can be used as a landmark for treatment as well.
- Downtime is minimal, typically 2 to 6 days, depending on the procedure.

INTRODUCTION

When topical options for axillary hyperhidrosis (HH) have failed, botulinum toxin is an effective, safe, and well-tolerated, although temporary, treatment option. For long-lasting or permanent efficacy, some patients turn to local procedures, such as superficial liposuction or manual curettage, or more invasive local surgery. Local surgical treatment is divided into 3 categories: (1) excision of skin and glandular tissue, (2) curettage or liposuction procedures to remove the subcutaneous sweat glands, or (3) a combination of limited skin excision with glandular tissue removal.[1] Complete skin excision is performed infrequently, because improved minimally invasive surgical techniques have become effective with fewer long-term complications.[2] The nonresponder rate varies from 2% to 20% with minimally invasive surgery and is likely the result of inadequate mapping of the hyperhidrotic area or inadequate surgical technique.[2] Newer, minimally invasive treatments have become available, such as microwave energy thermolysis.

PATIENT EVALUATION OVERVIEW

A thorough HH history should be obtained from the patient, including age of onset of HH, location and symmetry of sweating, aggravating/alleviating factors, previous treatments for HH, family history of HH, and current medications that may exacerbate the condition. A physical examination should be performed to rule out a possible secondary cause of HH that needs to be treated. A starch-iodine test is then performed to identify the dimensions of the involved area for treatment. The Minor starch-iodine test is a cheap and

Disclosure: D.A. Glaser has served as advisor for Allergan, Galderma, Miramar Labs, and Unilever. She has been an investigator and received research grants from Allergan, Miramar Labs, and Ulthera. T.A. Galperin has nothing to disclose.
Department of Dermatology, Saint Louis University School of Medicine, 1402 South Grand Boulevard-ABI, St Louis, MO 63104, USA
* Corresponding author.
E-mail address: glasermd@slu.edu

Dermatol Clin 32 (2014) 533–540
http://dx.doi.org/10.1016/j.det.2014.06.014

simple procedure commonly used to detect focal areas of sweating. The affected area is first dried, then an iodine solution is brushed onto the skin and allowed to dry. A starch powder, such as corn starch, is peppered on top, and the area is observed for a few minutes. Purple-black dots develop when sweat interacts with the starch and iodine. If a positive starch-iodine test cannot be obtained, the hair-bearing portion of the axilla should be treated.

The amount of axillary sweating can be assessed using the patient-reported Hyperhidrosis Disease Severity Scale (HDSS) (**Table 1**). The HDSS can also be obtained during the postoperative period to assess treatment success. Gravimetric (weight-based) assessment is an objective measurement typically performed in research studies but is not practical for routine clinical use.

In addition, surgical risks need to be ascertained before considering which procedure may be best suited for the patient. Antiplatelet therapies and bleeding diathesis are relative contraindications. Patients with significant arthritis or previous injury to the shoulder area may limit access to the axillary vault for certain procedures, and pain in the area may limit the patient's ability to maintain proper arm position during surgery, even if good range of motion is present.

MANAGEMENT GOALS

The goals of therapy are to provide a permanent or long-lasting solution for axillary HH, with a minimally invasive procedure that is cost-effective, easily accessible, and has minimal side effects and downtime.

SURGICAL TREATMENT OPTIONS AND PROCEDURE
Excision

Surgical excision can either be a radical excision of the skin and glandular tissue (RSE) (ie, en bloc

resection), or a limited skin excision with glandular tissue removal (LSE), such as the modified Shelley procedure. Surgical complication rates from RSE are high, and the procedure is rarely performed.[1] The relapse rate can vary. A study of 125 patients[3] undergoing LSE found a 12.8% relapse rate.

RSE can be performed via several different surgical techniques, each differing in the method of axillary skin removal and type of wound closure.[4] RSE can be performed under tumescent anesthesia, and the wounds sutured, generally requiring a subcutaneous drain for 1 to 2 days after treatment.[4]

Excessive sweating, as measured by gravimetric assessment, at 12 months after treatment is reduced by about 65%.[4] In studies, the average aesthetic outcome reported by patients was graded as moderate. Side effects of treatment include hematoma formation (20%), paresthesia (33.3%), focal alopecia (100%), and skin infection (13%).[4] Poor aesthetic outcomes, with scarring and skin retraction, which can lead to a decreased range of motion of the shoulder,[5] and long recovery times are 2 reasons that en bloc resections are rarely, if ever, performed.

With the skin-sparing technique (LSE), surgeons can perform the procedure on 1 axilla at a treatment session,[1,3] or both axillae can be treated simultaneously.[4] Antibiotic prophylaxis can be given an hour before the procedure, if deemed necessary. The area of maximal sweating is identified via the Minor starch-iodine test, and then, the axilla is anesthetized with lidocaine 1% and epinephrine 1:100,000[1] or tumescent anesthesia.[4] The elliptical area of maximal sweating, approximately 4 cm × 1 cm in diameter (horizontally), is excised down to the subcutaneous fat. The adjacent hair-bearing area of excessive sweating is undermined with Metzenbaum scissors to the affected edges, and the wound edges are everted to expose the 1-mm to 2-mm pink, papular sweat glands adhering to the dermis.[1] Sweat glands are cut out with curved scissors to defat the dermis, and the wound is closed with sutures. A subcutaneous drain is required for 1 to 2 days after treatment. A figure-of-eight dressing is applied for 10 days,[4] or a compression dressing for 24 hours.[3]

Excessive sweating, as measured by gravimetric assessment, at 12 months after treatment was reduced by a mean of 63% in 1 case series.[4] An early case series,[1] using a subjective, patient-assessed measure of sweat reduction after treatment, found a mean sweat reduction of 65%. The average aesthetic outcome reported by patients was graded as good,[4] 58.4% of patients

Table 1 HDSS	
How Would You Rate the Severity of Your Hyperhidrosis?	
HDSS Score	**Definition**
1	Never noticeable, never interferes
2	Tolerable, sometimes interferes
3	Barely tolerable, frequently interferes
4	Intolerable and always interferes

were satisfied with treatment, and 82.4% would choose the same procedure again.[3] The mean amount of time to return to work is reported to vary from 4 to 8.8 days.[1,3]

Side effects and scarring are less prevalent than with en bloc excision. The mean scar length is 5 cm, and scar formation does not lead to functional impairment, compared with a scar length of 9.3 cm, and a relatively high prevalence of functional impairment in the RSE group.[3,4] Side effects include hematoma formation (18.2%), paresthesia (27.3%), focal alopecia (100%), seroma formation (27.3%), fibrotic bridles (27.3%), skin erosion (36.4%), skin infection (5.6%), hypertrophic scarring (13/99), and flap necrosis (18.2%).[3,4]

Liposuction

Because the eccrine glands are located at the superficial subcutaneous plane, liposuction procedures have been used to remove the sweat glands without having to excise tissue. Liposuction has been used safely, and with moderate long-term efficacy in axillary HH. Patients can receive antibiotic prophylaxis with ciprofloxacin 500 mg orally × 1 dose an hour before the procedure,[6] although most physicians do not pretreat with antibiotics. Like other procedures, a starch-iodine test is helpful to identify the area of HH. Two small incisions are made in the superior and inferior borders of the axilla to deliver tumescent anesthesia. Once the skin is visibly blanched, the suction cannula is used to superficially remove the subcutaneous fat. Physicians have a variety of cannulas to choose from (**Fig. 1**), but in general, the more aggressive cannulas provide greater reduction of sweat, although they may be associated with

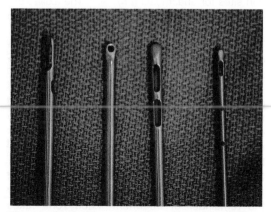

Fig. 1. Liposuction cannulas showing different configurations.

higher risks of adverse events.[6] The hole of the cannula is oriented toward the skin surface, and the sweat glands are scraped away from the underside of the dermis using a back-and-forth motion in a crisscross pattern.[7,8] Incisions are generally not closed, but are left open for drainage. A compression bandage can be applied for 24 hours.[6,7]

In 1 study comparing 3 different cannulas,[6] the investigators found a 44% and 49% reduction in sweating, obtained by gravimetric measurements, with a 1-hole and 3-hole cannula, respectively. The relapse rate with liposuction can be as high as 40% several months after treatment.[7] Side effects are minor and temporary. They include bruising, hematoma formation (43%), skin erosion (7%–14%), bridle formation (21%), paresthesia (43%–50%), and partial alopecia (14%).[6,8]

Liposuction-Curettage

Liposuction-curettage (LC) has been safely and effectively performed for many years. There are several different treatment techniques, which differ in their type and size of incisions, type of cannula and curette used, and the aggressiveness of the procedure. The experience of the surgeon is also an important factor. Tumescent anesthesia is administered, and small incisions are made into the central and upper inner axilla.[3,4,9] Alternatively, a modified technique can be used, in which 4 or 5 2-mm, evenly spaced, vertically oriented incisions are made using a punch biopsy instrument 1 cm beyond the lateral margin of the axilla, and 4 or 5 similarly sized and spaced incisions are made horizontally 1 cm beyond the inferior margin.[10] LC is performed using a liposuction device and a sharp, rasping-type cannula applied to the dermal-subcutaneous interface. Blunt cannulas may not remove sweat glands as proficiently as cannulas with curettage.[3,4,9] Back-and-forth strokes are performed with an upward tension, and the surgeon's thumb and forefinger provide pressure on the skin at either end of the cannula.[4,10]

Intraoperative indicators of sufficient LC include a complete elevation of the skin from subcutaneous fat, lividity of the skin, and no fat adhering to the dermis.[9,10] Incisions are closed with either Steri-Strips™ (3M, St. Paul, MN) or sutures but can be left open for better drainage. A compression bandage for 24 hours or a figure-of-eight dressing for 10 days is applied.[3,4]

Excessive sweating, as measured by gravimetric assessment, at 6 to 12 months after treatment, can be reduced by 60.4% to 69% in 89% to 93% of patients.[4,6,10] The mean HDSS score of 3.05 decreased to 2.75 6 months after treatment, which was statistically significant.[10] The aesthetic outcome reported by patients was graded as either very good or good,[4] and 78.4% to 84% of patients were completely satisfied or satisfied with the procedure[3,4,9]; 94.6% of patients would choose the same procedure again.[3] The relapse rate is approximately 14.5%, and the mean amount of time to return to work was only 1.3 days.[3]

Side effects of treatment are mild and temporary, and include hematoma formation (20%–78.4%), paresthesia (11.8%–26.7%), focal alopecia (7.8%–60%), seroma formation (6.7%–13.7%), skin erosion (20%–32%), bridle formation (10.8%–53.3%), and flap necrosis (6.7%).[3,4,9] There is only a small risk of skin infection. Skin ulceration and full-thickness skin necrosis can occur with aggressive LC, without any added efficacy.[11] Scarring is minimal, with the average scar length of 1 cm, and without hypertrophy or functional impairment.[3,4]

The exact duration of efficacy of LC is difficult to ascertain, because past studies had many variations in surgical expertise, surgical techniques, methods of measuring efficacy, and no consistent follow-up of patients past 1 year.

Curettage

There are several different treatment techniques, which differ in their type and size of incisions, type of cannula and curette used, and the aggressiveness of the procedure. Tumescent anesthesia is used, followed by a 2-cm to 3-cm incision made caudally from the marked zone,[12] or 2 or 3 5-mm incisions can be made at the margins of the axillae.[13] The marked area is undermined using Metzenbaum scissors, and a sharp, gynecologic[12] or number 2 curette[13] is used within the dermis. After curettage, the wound is closed with subcutaneous and superficial sutures, and a suction drained is placed within the axilla until secretions are lower than 10 mL/d.[12] Conversely, with 2 or 3 small incisions, wounds can be closed with adhesive strips, and a compression bandage applied for 24 hours.[13]

At 6 months after treatment, 36.4% of patients had a very good outcome, and 29.9% of patients had a good outcome, based on subjective assessment.[12] Excessive sweating, as measured by gravimetric assessment, at a median 11 months after treatment can be reduced by more than 50% in 93% of patients[13]; 90.9% of patients would recommend the procedure to others.[12] The relapse rate with this procedure is approximately 29%.[13]

Side effects include infection (2.2%), epidermal necrosis (2.2%), hematoma formation (13.3%), a markedly visible scar (27%), paresthesia (33%), partial alopecia (44%), hyperpigmentation (33%), and skin ulceration (12%).[12,13]

MiraDry

The MiraDry device is a new, nonsurgical treatment that is cleared by the US Food and Drug Administration (FDA) for axillary HH. It uses microwave energy to destroy eccrine sweat glands. Microwave energy is preferentially absorbed by tissue with a high water content, such as the sweat glands. The microwave energy leads to rapid molecular rotation, which generates frictional heat and cellular thermolysis.[14,15]

The device consists of a console, a handpiece, and a single-use biotip (**Fig. 2**). The antennae, within the handpiece, focus microwave energy on to the dermal-adipose interface, regardless of skin thickness.[14,15] There is simultaneous cooling and monitoring of the skin temperature, during the energy cycle, to avert thermal transfer of heat into the epidermis. There are 5 energy settings, which regulate the duration and depth of heat to be delivered, and the vacuum system within the biotip helps to stabilize the skin during the treatment.[14]

A few days before the procedure, patients should shave their axillae, and 1 to 2 hours before the procedure, patients should take ibuprofen 800 mg to minimize posttreatment tenderness and edema. A starch-iodine test is performed to identify the area of prominent sweating, after this, the axillary vault is measured with a supplied grid. Alternatively, the hair-bearing skin can be treated. The grid measures the length and width of the vault in millimeters. A temporary template, fitting the specified measurements, is applied to the vault to identify the treatment zones and injection sites for anesthesia (**Fig. 3**).[14] The axillae are injected with lidocaine 1% and epinephrine 1:100,000, up to the maximum level of 7 mg/kg. The discomfort associated with lidocaine injection can be lessened by buffering the lidocaine with sodium bicarbonate.

The initial energy setting can be set to 1 (lowest), 2, or 3. We prefer to perform the initial treatment at level 3. The biotip automatically starts at the lowest energy setting in the upper inner axilla, where the skin is thinnest and the overlying nerves are closer to the skin surface. After the upper zones are treated, the energy level is automatically adjusted to the specified level for the remainder of treatment. Each zone takes approximately 45 seconds to treat (**Fig. 4**), and

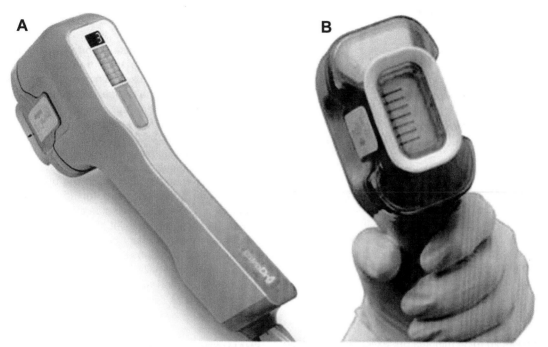

Fig. 2. (*A, B*) Handpiece and single-use biotip used for microwave thermolysis. (*Courtesy of* Miramar Labs, Santa Clara, CA; with permission.)

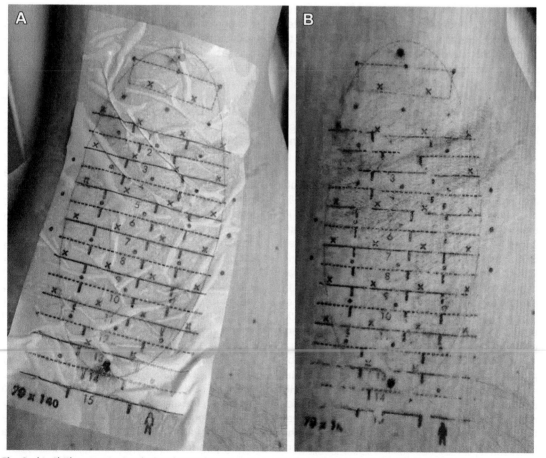

Fig. 3. (*A, B*) The appropriately sized template is placed onto the axillary vault. Alcohol is dabbed on to the tissue to transfer the template pattern to the axilla.

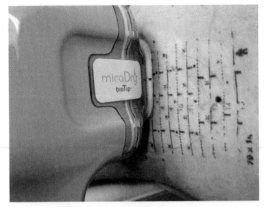

Fig. 4. As each zone is treated, cooling plates in the biotip cool the epidermis. (*Courtesy of* Miramar Labs, Santa Clara, CA; with permission.)

1-point to 3-point decrease reported by the patients. The investigators have treated a limited number of patients whose main complaint is axillary body odor with the device, and patients have described improvement, but clearly more studies are needed.

Common and minor side effects include edema, redness from vacuum suction, and axillary tenderness/pain for several days' duration.[16] Altered sensation (numbness, tingling) in the upper arm or axilla can occur and lasts for approximately 5 weeks.[16,17] Less common side effects reported include blisters or burns at the treatment site, skin irritation/rash, axillary bumps, patchy alopecia, and mild compensatory sweating.[16,17] Patients can occasionally have edema outside the treatment area, and rarely, they can have temporary nerve injury.

it takes 20 to 30 minutes per axilla, depending on the axilla size and energy level. After the treatment, patients are given an ice pack wrapped in gauze or a paper towel and instructed to keep it in place for 15 to 20 minutes at a time every 1 to 2 hours, for the first 48 hours after treatment. Patients are also instructed to continue nonsteroidal antiinflammatory agents such as ibuprofen 400 mg every 4 to 6 hours for the first 48 hours. Patients require 2 treatment sessions, with a second treatment performed 3 months after the initial one.[16] The treatment delay allows time for healing and fibrosis, which further reduces the number of eccrine and apocrine glands.[16,17] Rarely, a third treatment is performed to achieve the desired outcome.

MiraDry is effective in reducing excess sweating. From the baseline HDSS assessment, 94% of patients experienced a 1-point decrease in their HDSS score,[16] and 55% to 83.3% experienced a 2-point or greater decrease in their HDSS score at 12 months after treatment.[16,18] Based on gravimetric assessments, 90% of patients experienced a 50% or greater reduction in axillary sweating, with an average reduction of 81.7%.[16] At 12 months after treatment, 85.5% of patients were satisfied with their treatment outcome.[16]

Improvement of axillary odor has been noted by patients.[18] Lee and colleagues reported using the microwave device on 11 Asian patients: 3 with HH only, 3 with HH and osmidrosis, and 5 with osmidrosis alone. The HDSS scores improved in all patients with HH (1-point to 3-point decrease in the HDSS) and axillary odor improved in all patient with osmidrosis. The improvement in odor was subjective and rated on a 4-point scale, with a

EVALUATION OF OUTCOME, ADJUSTMENT OF TREATMENT, AND LONG-TERM RECOMMENDATIONS

To our knowledge, there are only a few randomized controlled trials comparing the efficacy of 2 procedures concurrently, which makes it difficult to assess the relative benefit of 1 procedure over another. A single randomized trial[4] compared the effectiveness, both histologically and gravimetrically, of RSE, LSE, and LC. The results showed that all 3 treatments had similar efficacy (minor differences were not statistically significant), but LC had the least amount of side effects, minimal scarring, and the least amount of down time. A randomized trial comparing LC versus curettage alone[19] found LC to be more effective, and with a similar side effect profile. Based on the available patient outcomes data, LC is the single best minimally invasive surgical treatment of axillary HH, in terms of efficacy, aesthetic outcome, and side effect profile.

The risk profile for RSE procedures does not justify their use, and procedures such as LC should be performed only by experienced surgeons, because the efficacy and safety of such procedures are operator dependent.

Since the initial advent of the invasive and minimally invasive surgical procedures for axillary HH, safer alternative treatments have become available, such as microwave thermolysis. When comparing the effectiveness, side effects, and patient satisfaction of the current procedural treatments for axillary HH (**Table 2**), microwave thermolysis may be the best available procedural treatment option, if the patient prefers a long-term solution.

Table 2
A comparison of the invasive and minimally invasive procedures for axillary HH

Procedure	Mean Reduction in HDSS	Mean Reduction with Gravimetric Measurements (%)	Mean Patient-Rated Satisfaction (%)	Mean Relapse Rate (%)	Common Side Effects (Mean %)	Less Common Side Effects (Mean %)
Liposuction	—	46.5	—	40	Bruising, hematoma formation (43), bridle formation (21), paresthesia (46.5)	Skin erosion (10.5), partial alopecia (14)
LC	0.30-point reduction	66	82.1 completely satisfied or satisfied	14.5	Paresthesia (19.8), hematoma (49.2), skin erosion (26.5), alopecia (33.9), bridle formation (29.3)	Flap necrosis (6.7), seroma formation (12.5), wound infection
Curettage	—	50	—	29	Hematoma (13.3), markedly visible scar (27), paresthesia (33), partial alopecia (44), hyperpigmentation (33)	Wound infection (2.2), epidermal necrosis (2.2), skin ulceration (12)
RSE	—	65.3	—	—	Hematoma (20), paresthesia (33.3), alopecia (100), large scar (100)	Wound infection (13)
LSE	—	62.9	58.4 satisfied	12.8	Hematoma (18.2), paresthesia (27.3), alopecia (100), seroma formation (27.3), bridle formation (27.3), skin erosion (36.4), flap necrosis (18.2)	Wound infection (5.6)
MiraDry	94 had a 1-point reduction	81.7	85.5 satisfied	—	Edema/erythema (90), paresthesia (65), patchy alopecia (26)	Blister formation (4.9), skin irritation (4.9), axillary bumps (2.5), mild compensatory sweating (2.5)

SUMMARY

Patients prefer treatments that are least invasive, require minimal downtime, and have good cosmetic results. Surgical treatments are effective at reducing excessive sweating, but require time for recovery after procedure, are operator dependent, and can have poor cosmetic outcomes. Treatment with microwave thermolysis is effective, minimally invasive, requires limited downtime, and has good cosmetic outcomes. Microwave thermolysis is the best minimally invasive procedural treatment of axillary HH and is FDA-cleared for such treatment. Other newer minimally invasive technologies are forthcoming, such as focused ultrasonography and fractional microneedle radiofrequency, which could prove to be efficacious as well.

REFERENCES

1. Lawrence CM, Lonsdale Eccles AA. Selective sweat gland removal with minimal skin excision in the treatment of axillary hyperhidrosis: a retrospective clinical and histological review of 15 patients. Br J Dermatol 2006;155(1):115–8. http://dx.doi.org/10.1111/j.1365-2133.2006.07320.x.

2. Bechara FG, Sand M, Altmeyer P. Characteristics of refractory sweating areas following minimally invasive surgery for axillary hyperhidrosis. Aesthetic Plast Surg 2008;33(3):308–11. http://dx.doi.org/10.1007/s00266-008-9261-4.

3. Wollina U, Köstler E, Schönlebe J, et al. Tumescent suction curettage versus minimal skin resection with subcutaneous curettage of sweat glands in axillary hyperhidrosis. Dermatol Surg 2008;34(5):709–16. http://dx.doi.org/10.1111/j.1524-4725.2008.34132.x.

4. Bechara FG, Sand M, Hoffmann K, et al. Histological and clinical findings in different surgical strategies for focal axillary hyperhidrosis: histologic and clinical findings. Dermatol Surg 2008;34(8):1001–9. http://dx.doi.org/10.1111/j.1524-4725.2008.34198.x.

5. Connolly M, de Berker D. Management of primary hyperhidrosis: a summary of the different treatment modalities. Am J Clin Dermatol 2003;4(10):681–97.

6. Bechara FG, Sand M, Sand D, et al. Surgical treatment of axillary hyperhidrosis: a study comparing liposuction cannulas with a suction-curettage cannula. Ann Plast Surg 2006;56(6):654–7. http://dx.doi.org/10.1097/01.sap.0000205771.40918.b3.

7. Lee MR, Ryman WJ. Liposuction for axillary hyperhidrosis. Australas J Dermatol 2005;46(2):76–9.

8. Swinehart JM. Treatment of axillary hyperhidrosis: combination of the starch-iodine test with the tumescent liposuction technique. Dermatol Surg 2000;26(4):392–6.

9. Bechara FG, Sand M, Tomi NS, et al. Repeat liposuction-curettage treatment of axillary hyperhidrosis is safe and effective. Br J Dermatol 2007;157(4):739–43. http://dx.doi.org/10.1111/j.1365-2133.2007.08092.x.

10. Ibrahim O, Kakar R, Bolotin D, et al. The comparative effectiveness of suction-curettage and onabotulinumtoxin-A injections for the treatment of primary focal axillary hyperhidrosis: a randomized control trial. J Am Acad Dermatol 2013;69(1):88–95. http://dx.doi.org/10.1016/j.jaad.2013.02.013.

11. Bechara FG, Sand M, Hoffmann K, et al. Aggressive shaving after combined liposuction and curettage for axillary hyperhidrosis leads to more complications without further benefit. Dermatol Surg 2008;34(7):952–3. http://dx.doi.org/10.1111/j.1524-4725.2008.34185.x.

12. Rompel R, Scholz S. Subcutaneous curettage vs. injection of botulinum toxin A for treatment of axillary hyperhidrosis. J Eur Acad Dermatol Venereol 2001;15(3):207–11.

13. Proebstle TM, Schneiders V, Knop J. Gravimetrically controlled efficacy of subcorial curettage: a prospective study for treatment of axillary hyperhidrosis. Dermatol Surg 2002;28(11):1022–6.

14. Jacob C. Treatment of hyperhidrosis with microwave technology. Semin Cutan Med Surg 2013;32(1):2–8.

15. Johnson JE, O'Shaughnessy KF, Kim S. Microwave thermolysis of sweat glands. Lasers Surg Med 2012;44(1):20–5. http://dx.doi.org/10.1002/lsm.21142.

16. Chih-Ho Hong H, Lupin M, O'Shaughnessy KF. Clinical evaluation of a microwave device for treating axillary hyperhidrosis. Dermatol Surg 2012;38(5):728–35. http://dx.doi.org/10.1111/j.1524-4725.2012.02375.x.

17. Glaser DA, Coleman WP, Fan LK, et al. A randomized, blinded clinical evaluation of a novel microwave device for treating axillary hyperhidrosis: the dermatologic reduction in underarm perspiration study. Dermatol Surg 2012;38(2):185–91. http://dx.doi.org/10.1111/j.1524-4725.2011.02250.x.

18. Lee SJ, Chang KY, Suh DH, et al. The efficacy of a microwave device for treating axillary hyperhidrosis and osmidrosis in Asians: a preliminary study. J Cosmet Laser Ther 2013;15(5):255–9. http://dx.doi.org/10.3109/14764172.2013.807114.

19. Tronstad C, Helsing P, Tønseth KA, et al. Tumescent suction curettage vs. curettage only for treatment of axillary hyperhidrosis evaluated by subjective and new objective methods. Acta Derm Venereol 2013;94(2):215–20. http://dx.doi.org/10.2340/00015555-1671.

Endoscopic Thoracic Sympathectomy

Eleni Moraites, MD[a], Olushola Akinshemoyin Vaughn, BA[b], Samantha Hill, MD[c],*

KEYWORDS

- Hyperhidrosis • Endoscopic thoracic sympathectomy • Palmar hyperhidrosis
- Axillary hyperhidrosis • Quality of life

KEY POINTS

- Endoscopic thoracic sympathectomy is a useful surgical approach in the treatment of selected patients with severe palmar hyperhidrosis.
- Approaches used to interrupt the sympathetic signal to the sweat glands include cutting or clipping the sympathetic chain.
- Ideal candidates for endoscopic thoracic sympathectomy are patients with onset before 16 years of age who are younger than 25 years at time of surgery, have body mass index less than 28, report no sweating during sleep, and have no significant comorbidities.
- Patients should be informed that endoscopic thoracic sympathectomy is associated with a high rate of the development of compensatory hyperhidrosis and that reversal procedures are unlikely to improve compensatory sweating.

INTRODUCTION AND HISTORY

The sympathectomy, a surgical procedure creating a break in the sympathetic signaling pathway, was pioneered in 1889 and at the time was used to treat conditions such as epilepsy, exophthalmic goiter, idiocy, and glaucoma. Although no longer indicated to treat these conditions, more advanced versions of the sympathectomy have found a place in the treatment of hyperhidrosis.[1] Hyperhidrosis is a skin disorder characterized by sweating in excess of what is necessary for thermoregulation of the body. This excessive sweating often involves the craniofacial region, axillae, palms, or soles and can be classified as either primary, which is idiopathic, or secondary to a medical condition or medication. Hyperhidrosis can be further classified as focal, regional, or generalized, with most patients suffering from primary focal hyperhidrosis. Various treatment modalities for the condition exist, including localized topical and injectable treatments, systemic medical treatments, and several surgical treatments.[2] The focus of this article is endoscopic thoracic sympathectomy (ETS) as management for primary focal hyperhidrosis.

Today the main indications for the sympathectomy are blushing, flushing, and hyperhidrosis.[1] Because hyperhidrosis is thought to potentially be caused by excessive sympathetic stimulation, the intention of ETS is to interrupt that signal by cutting or clipping the involved sympathetic nerves.[2] The procedure is noted to have particular success in the improvement of palmar hyperhidrosis.[3] Initially, the sympathectomy was an open procedure, but it has evolved into an endoscopic surgical technique.[1] The main goal over time has been to maintain efficacy while minimizing the invasiveness of the procedure in an effort to reduce the

Financial Disclosures: There are no financial disclosures to report for any of the authors.
[a] Hennepin County Medical Center, 701 Park Avenue, Minneapolis, MN 55415, USA; [b] School of Medicine and Public Health, University of Wisconsin-Madison, 750 Highland Avenue, Madison, WI 53705, USA; [c] RidgeView Dermatology, 101 Candlewood Court, Lynchburg, VA 24502, USA
* Corresponding author.
E-mail addresses: hillsa1@gmail.com; sehill@ridgeviewdermatology.com

derm.theclinics.com

risk of complications, specifically the development of compensatory sweating.[1,4]

ANATOMY AND PHYSIOLOGY

The sympathetic nerves that control sweating originate in the spinal cord between segments T1 and L2. The distribution is segmental and variable, with sympathetic fibers from T1 generally supplying the head, T2 the neck, T3 to T6 the thorax, T7 to T11 the abdomen, and T12 to L2 the legs.[5,6]

Experiments performed in the 1950s found that most of the sympathetic outflow to the hand originates from T2 to T3.[7] Signaling from these levels may also travel via an alternative pathway, the nerve of Kuntz. Although not present in all people, the nerve of Kuntz forms a connection from the second intercostal nerve to the first thoracic ventral ramus, allowing signals to reach the brachial plexus without traversing the sympathetic trunk.[8] Therefore, complete denervation of the hand requires surgical division of the sympathetic chain above the T2 ganglion and below the T3 ganglion as well as possible transection of Kuntz's nerve.[5] When axillary hyperhidrosis exists with palmar hyperhidrosis, surgery may be extended to include the T4, T5, or even T6 ganglion.[6,9] The cervicothoracic ganglion, or stellate ganglion, is formed by the fusion of the inferior cervical ganglion and the first thoracic ganglion. It has been implicated in hyperhidrosis but is often left untouched during ETS to avoid Horner's syndrome.[10] More specific information regarding these techniques will be addressed in a later section of this review.

Endoscopic lumbar sympathectomy is has been used for plantar hyperhidrosis. Sympathetic outflow to the lower extremities originates at T12, L1, and L2 and, therefore, can be interrupted by division of the sympathetic trunk at the L3 level or removal of the ganglia from L2 to L4.[6] In surgery, the first lumbar ganglion often is left untouched in an attempt to preserve sexual function.[6]

NOMENCLATURE

Various terms have been used to describe origins of sympathetic innervation with regard to the exact location of surgical intervention. Some authors describe the vertebral level (T), whereas others describe sympathetic outflow by its relationship with the nearest rib (R). Recently, the International Society on Sympathetic Surgery and The Society of Thoracic Surgeons General Thoracic Task Force on Hyperhidrosis acknowledged the need for uniform language to describe the location of ETS in an effort to make comparisons between procedures more accurate.[2] A consensus on terminology, as determined by International Society on Sympathetic Surgery and the Society of Thoracic Surgeons in 2011, indicates that standard nomenclature using rib orientation is the most precise way to describe ETS. An operative note would describe the procedure by noting the rib number (for example, R3 is the third rib) and the location (top, bottom, or both) where the denervation occurred relative to the rib.[2] For example, a procedure at R4, above denotes nerve interruption above the fourth rib. Both R and T nomenclature, including the use of R nomenclature without the denotation of above and below, are used in the literature and are so used in this report.

INDICATIONS

Referral for ETS may be indicated when medical therapies and, when appropriate, local surgery have failed or are contraindicated. Other treatments for axillary hyperhidrosis include topical antiperspirants such as aluminum chloride; injected botulinum toxin; oral anticholinergic medications; and local surgeries including simple excision, curettage, and liposuction and procedures that combine these techniques.[9] More recently, microwave and ultrasound technologies have also been used to treat axillary hyperhidrosis. For palmar hyperhidrosis, standard treatments include topical aluminum chloride, oral anticholinergic medications, iontophoresis, and botulinum toxin. For craniofacial hyperhidrosis, treatments include topical aluminum chloride, botulinum toxin, and oral medications such as anticholinergics, clonidine, propranolol, and diltiazem.[9,11] The algorithm for treatment strategies in plantar hyperhidrosis is similar to that of palmar hyperhidrosis, with ultimate referral for endoscopic lumbar sympathectomy rather than thoracic sympathectomy.[9,12]

Based on randomized trials and nonrandomized comparisons, the Society of Thoracic Surgeons has described an ideal candidate for ETS[2]:

- Patients with onset before 16 years of age who are younger than 25 years at time of surgery
  - with body mass index less than 28
  - reporting no sweating during sleep
  - without significant comorbidities and
  - with resting heart rate greater than 55 beats per minute.

Additional indications for ETS include[1]:

- Arteriospastic disorders: eg, Raynaud's disease and acrocyanosis
- Occlusive arteriolar disorders: eg, thrombongiitis obliterans

- Some neurologic disorders: eg, posttraumatic sympathetic dystrophy
- Intractable pain: eg, angina and complex regional pain syndrome
- Possibly social phobia

Selection criteria for randomized trials exploring surgical treatment of hyperhidrosis frequently include only severe and debilitating primary palmar hyperhidrosis with serious negative repercussions on social life and professional activity.[13,14] According to the Society of Thoracic Surgeons Expert Consensus, "only a small percentage of patients should be considered for surgical treatment."[2]

TECHNIQUES

The goal of a sympathectomy of any kind for hyperhidrosis is to disconnect the eccrine sweat glands from the sympathetic signals that trigger them to initiate sweating. Initially, open procedures were performed, with approaches including anterior supraclavicular, posterior paravertebral, posterior midline, anterior thoracic, axillary thoracic, or axillary extrathoracic with first rib resection.[15] In 1951, Kux first described an endoscopic transthoracic approach, and this technique is now the standard of care for hyperhidrosis.[4]

Current techniques involve the destruction of the bilateral thoracic sympathetic ganglia via endoscopic resection, ablation, or clipping (**Fig. 1**).[2,16] The procedure requires general anesthesia, but most patients are able to go home the day of the procedure. There are reports of the use of local anesthesia for the procedure, but this is not generally recommended.[2,16]

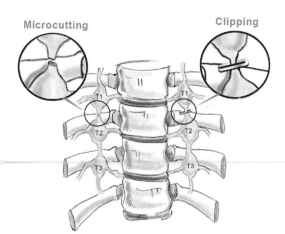

Fig. 1. Current techniques for endoscopic thoracic sympathectomy. (*Courtesy of* Albert Ganss, International Hyperhidrosis Society, Quakertown, PA; with permission.)

Surgical technique can vary based on surgeon preference and anatomic location of hyperhidrosis. Recent consensus recommendations from the Society of Thoracic Surgeons are to interrupt the sympathetic chain above the third rib for palmar hyperhidrosis, above the fourth and fifth rib for axillary hyperhidrosis, and above the third rib for craniofacial hyperhidrosis (**Table 1**).[2]

Traditionally, for isolated palmar hyperhidrosis, an incision of less than 1 cm is made in the midaxillary line, through which the endoscope and instruments are inserted. Carbon dioxide insufflation may be used to partially collapse the lung, improving visualization. The anatomy is examined, and the sympathetic chain is divided, often just above T2 and below the stellate ganglion.[4,17] Additional sites may be interrupted, including other ganglia and nerves of Kuntz if present. The ends of the nerves are separated to allow at least a 1-cm gap to reduce nerve regrowth and recurrence of hyperhidrosis. Sympathetic tone to the hand is assessed with a laser Doppler palmar blood flow device or finger temperature probe. A suction catheter is used to evacuate the pneumothorax if the lung has been collapsed; otherwise, intrapleural air is aspirated through tubes. A chest x-ray is obtained after the procedure to ensure proper lung inflation and minimal intrapleural air. The procedure generally takes less than an hour to complete.[4,17]

Researchers have attempted to analyze whether transection, resection, ablation, or clipping is a superior technique in ETS. No clear differences have been found.[2,18] Rather, the results are dependent on whether the correct level of division was achieved and if there was enough separation between the ends of the chain to avoid nerve regrowth.[2]

A few small prospective studies out of China have recently found an effective new technique using a transumbilical endoscopic approach to achieve thoracic sympathectomy. In one study,

Table 1 Society of Thoracic Surgeons consensus	
Location of Hyperhidrosis	Recommended Surgical Level
Palmar hyperhidrosis	Above third rib (driest palms) or above fourth rib (palms less dry but reduced chance of compensatory sweating)
Axillary hyperhidrosis	Above fourth and fifth rib
Craniofacial hyperhidrosis	Above third rib

66 patients with severe palmar hyperhidrosis presented for thoracic sympathectomy.[19] Thirty-four of these patients received transumbilical thoracic sympathectomies through a 5-mm umbilical incision using an ultrathin gastroscope; the remaining patients were treated with traditional needlescopic thoracic sympathectomy.[19] All of the patients reported that the procedure successfully treated their hyperhidrosis. Patients receiving the transumbilical procedure reported reduced pain and paresthesia; this is possibly explained by the absence of a chest wall incision and subsequent lack of manipulation of intercostal space with trocars. This transumbilical technique showed a superior aesthetic outcome when compared with the traditional group, although the operating time of the surgery was slightly longer.[19]

Use of a voice-controlled robotic arm has been compared with use of a human camera-holding assistant.[20] There was no difference between groups in terms of accidents, pain, general satisfaction, anhidrosis, length of hospitalization, or compensatory hyperhidrosis (CH). The robotic group had reduced contact of the laparoscopic lens with mediastinal structures but also had longer operating time, suggesting that the robotic camera is as safe as a human assistant but less efficient.[20]

OUTCOMES

The ETS procedure is thought to relieve palmar hyperhidrosis in greater than 95% of patients.[21] Recurrent sweating develops in 0% to 65% of patients that undergo the procedure.[2] Compensatory sweating occurs in up to 98% of patients.[2] Patient satisfaction is reported to be between 66.7% and 93% but is known to decline with time.[22]

Four main studies show the trends in satisfaction and complication rates of ETS.

Unilateral or Bilateral ETS

A 1994 study followed up with 270 patients who had unilateral or bilateral ETS for upper extremity hyperhidrosis, with a total of 480 sympathectomies.[23] Patients who had undergone ETS between 1965 and 1992 were sent a questionnaire regarding early postoperative results, side effects, complications, and long-term effects of the procedure; the average time between the procedure and receipt of the questionnaire was 16.4 years, ranging from 9 months to 27.1 years.[23] Results from the questionnaire indicate treatment failure in 1.9% of cases and symptom recurrence in 1.5%. A total of 95.5% of patients were initially completely satisfied, 66.7% were completely satisfied at follow-up, and 26.7% were partially satisfied. Reported side effects include compensatory

sweating (67.4%), gustatory sweating (50.7%), severe dryness of the hands (<1.2%), and Horner's syndrome (2.5%).[23]

Bilateral ETS

In 1995, Drott and colleagues[24] followed up with 850 patients for 31 months after bilateral ETS for upper extremity hyperhidrosis. Treatment failure was reported in 2% of patients with symptom recurrence in 2% of patients. 98% reported satisfactory results at the end of follow-up. Compensatory sweating occurred in 55% of patients, with 2% considering this as disturbing as their original symptoms.[24] Gustatory sweating occurred in 36% of patients, but was often relieved with anticholinergic drugs and not considered a major problem by patients. The use of anticholinergic medications to treat other forms of compensatory sweating was not discussed. Three patients developed Horner's syndrome, one of which was temporary.[24]

More recently, a 2013 study followed up with 51 patients for up to 16 years.[25] The investigators reported treatment failure in 2% of patients; recurrence rate was not discussed. A total of 86.3% of patients rated their satisfaction as excellent or good, and 9.8% were not happy. Of the not happy, 3 suffered postoperative chest pain, one had a pneumothorax and empyema leading to prolonged hospital stay, and one had treatment failure.[25] A total of 97.4% of patients experienced compensatory sweating. Patients with compensatory sweating located on the back rather than face, axilla, abdomen, thighs, or feet were more likely to rate satisfaction as excellent or good.[25]

Gender Differences in Outcomes of ETS

Finally, a 2010 study analyzed gender differences in outcomes of ETS by surveying 1044 patients, 719 women and 325 men, who underwent surgery for palmar hyperhidrosis from 2000 to 2008.[26] Treatment failure was reported in 1.2% of patients, regardless of gender, but overall recurrence rate was not discussed. In a survey 30 days after surgery, there were no significant differences in quality of life reported between genders.[26] Overall, 95% of patients reported that their quality of life was either better or much better, and 1.5% claimed their quality of life was a little worse or much worse. Results indicating perceived postsurgical differences in quality of life were similar for both genders.[26]

Outcomes Variances

Outcomes are highly dependent on the level of interruption of the sympathetic chain. Recent literature compared multiple-level sympathectomy with single ganglia ETS. Meta-analysis suggests that there is no significant difference in efficacy between groups.[27] However, one study found that clipping above and below T4 improved efficacy and lowered the risk of compensatory sweating when compared with T2 to T4 sympathectomy.[28] For palmar hyperhidrosis, the Society of Thoracic Surgeons consensus document suggests that 2 interruptions are made, at R3 and R4, for patients who are willing to accept a higher risk of CH to have completely dry hands. R3 or R4 interruption alone may be appropriate to limit the likelihood of CH, although it may result in moister hands.[2]

Additional studies have sought to further compare the efficacy of single ganglia ETS at different levels for palmar hyperhidrosis, with one showing improved effectiveness at R3 (above the third rib, usually T3) when compared with R2 (above the second rib, usually R2). This study found that treatment failure was more common with R3 sympathecotomy, but the persistent palmar hyperhidrosis could be cured with reoperation at the R2 level.[29]

Finally, preoperative characteristics may be predictive of poor postoperative results. Younger age, male sex, and higher levels of preoperative and postoperative sweating may predict treatment failure, whereas increased age may correlate with increased CH after surgery.[29]

VARIATION IN OUTCOMES BY ANATOMIC LOCATION OF HYPERHIDROSIS

The outcomes of ETS vary based on the anatomic location of the sweating. Patients undergoing operation for palmar hyperhidrosis tend to be more satisfied than those with axillary hyperhidrosis, at 46.2% and 33.3% respectively.[23] Recurrence rates may be dramatically different between palmar and axillary hyperhidrosis, with one study finding recurrence rates of 6.6% for palmar hyperhidrosis and 65% for axillary.[30]

Patients with palmar hyperhidrosis often have concomitant plantar hyperhidrosis, so the optimal treatment strategy for patients with palmoplantar hyperhidrosis has been analyzed. In one study, 73 patients were treated for hyperhidrosis with an endoscopic thoracic sympathetic block, 66 of whom had both palmar and plantar hyperhidrosis. The study showed that 100% of patients had nearly or completely dry palms after an endoscopic thoracic sympathetic block with a clip placed at T4, and 50% of the patients showed relief from plantar sweating, although the mechanism for this improvement is unclear.[31] For patients with palmoplantar hyperhidrosis, additional

interruption at R5 may be superior to sympathectomy at R4 alone,[2] but some clinicians note that long-term results tend to be poor.[12] Plantar hyperhidrosis may be more tolerated than other forms of hyperhidrosis because excessive sweat on the feet is easier to conceal and is often considered more socially acceptable than excessive sweating in other areas of the body.

ETS is used for craniofacial hyperhidrosis in cases of clinical severity.[9] It is critical to distinguish isolated craniofacial hyperhidrosis from facial blushing. Facial blushing is best treated with T2 sympathectomy,[32] whereas craniofacial hyperhidrosis is best treated by R3-alone interruption.[2] By one analysis, patients with facial hyperhidrosis were more likely to be either satisfied or regret having the procedure as opposed to patients with facial blushing, who were most likely to say they were very satisfied after surgery. All patients in this study had ETS at R2, R2 to R3 or R2 to R4.[33]

COMPLICATIONS

ETS is an elective procedure that has great potential benefits but also some significant risks. Patients having this procedure are often greatly distressed by the social and occupational limitations that are often associated with hyperhidrosis and must be well informed before electing to have this procedure.[2] Also, because most patients that have this procedure are less than 30 years of age, it is important to consider that these individuals in whom complications do arise may have many years of suffering after the procedure.

Potential complications from ETS include[30,34–37]:

- Development of Horner's syndrome: 1%–2.5%
- Pneumothorax: 7%
- Hemothorax: 1%
- Paresthesia: up to 50%
- Compensatory sweating: >50%
- Hyperthermia
- Bradycardia requiring a pacemaker

A literature review of the complications of ETS was performed in 2004 looking for patterns of potentially significant drawbacks to having the procedure; this was a Medline search using terms "*thoracoscopic sympathectomy, endoscopic thoracic sympathectomy,*" and *complications.*[38] Results of the review show that the most common short-term complication of the procedure is a spontaneously resolving postoperative pneumothorax. Approximately 5% of patients have significant intrathoracic bleeding but only a minority will go on to require a thoracotomy to correct this problem. An extremely common long-term complication is compensatory sweating. Ojimba and Cameron[38] reported 1% to 2% of patients regretted having the procedure because of the severity of the compensatory sweating.

A more recent analysis of 1731 cases indicates that the most common immediate postoperative complication is pain (97.4%) and estimates the late complication of compensatory sweating at 88.4%.[39] Immediate postoperative complications also include pneumothorax (3.5%), neurologic disorders of the upper limbs (2.1%), Horner's syndrome (0.9%), significant bleeding (0.4%), and extensive subcutaneous emphysema.[39]

Although there are no published known deaths from ETS, anecdotally there are 9 known deaths after ETS resulting from severe hemorrhage or complications from anesthesia.[38]

COMPENSATORY SWEATING

Of all the known risks associated with ETS, it is perhaps most important for the patient to understand the risk of compensatory sweating. Compensatory sweating, also called compensatory hyperhidrosis (CH), occurs when treatment for hyperhidrosis decreases or eliminates sweating in the original problem area, but the body then compensates by increasing sweat production in another remote location.[2,38] CH is the most common side effect of ETS, and literature cites that CH develops in anywhere between 3% and 98% of patients.[2] This wide range may be accounted for by varying definitions of CH and variations in the surgical approach for treatment of hyperhidrosis. The most common sites for CH occurrence are abdomen, back, legs, and gluteal area.[40] Adult patients and those who have a preexisting tendency to sweat in the inguinal folds, buttocks, back, and upper thighs are at greater risk for CH.[2,41] Pediatric patients and those undergoing a single ganglion transection not involving T2 report the lowest rates of CH.[41]

Most studies do not quantify the level of severity of compensatory sweating, but a 2009 study sought to measure severity using patient questionnaires.[41] Severity was measured on a 10-point scale, with 10 being unbearable and 0 being no symptoms, and was assessed at each site of compensatory sweating. Overall, compensatory sweating rated 4.5 in severity and was most commonly found in the back, abdomen, chest, legs, and thighs. Age was the only independent predictor of CH in multivariate analysis, whereas age and multilevel sympathectomy were independent predictors of a high severity score. Operation on T2 and high severity score were independent predictors of patient dissatisfaction.[41]

The current trend with regard to limiting the possibility of compensatory sweating is performing a sympathectomy at T4 alone.[2,40] Several studies found that this technique may reduce the risk of compensatory sweating greatly. In one study of 276 patients with axillary hyperhidrosis, 78.3% underwent thermal ablation of T3/T4, whereas 21.7% had thermal ablation of T4 alone. The study indicated that the T4 group reported higher satisfaction rate, lower recurrence rate, and lower severity of compensatory sweating.[40] A meta-analysis of studies published in the last decade indicated that T3 sympathectomy is recommended for the treatment of palmar hyperhidrosis regardless of the surgical technique used.[27]

QUALITY OF LIFE

Although compensatory sweating may arise after ETS, it is important to determine if quality of life is improved regardless of complications. A 2012 study of the evolution of quality of life over 5 years in 453 patients who had ETS found that patients had immediate and sustained improvement in quality of life over the course of the study.[42] This was a prospective, nonrandomized and uncontrolled study carried out via questionnaire regarding quality of life following ETS. The questionnaire was given perioperatively, at 30 days, and at 5 years after the procedure. The study found that 97.3% of patients had complete remission of palmar, axillary, or facial sweating after 5 years. Those who did have an improvement in quality of life from ETS had sustained improvement over 5 years. Although 71.5% of patients reported moderate-to-severe compensatory sweating, only 1.5% of patients were dissatisfied with the results of the procedure.[42]

The factor that most influences postsurgical quality of life is compensatory sweating. Therefore, patients should be informed of this side effect, and treatment should be tailored to reduce compensatory sweating based on anatomic location and patient preferences.[2,43] In general, higher levels of blockade on the sympathetic chain correspond to higher regret rates. Patients should also be made aware that the most satisfied patients are those with palmar or palmar-axillary hyperhidrosis, or both.[2] Another significant factor is the recurrence of symptoms after ETS. Recurrence of hyperhidrosis after surgery has been reported with incidence of between 0% and 65%; the variability may be explained by use of different surgical techniques, level of sympathetic interruption, and durations of follow-up care.[2] If recurrence of hyperhidrosis occurs, it usually recurs within 18 months of surgery.[21]

REVERSAL

In some instances, the CH after ETS is severe enough to warrant attempt at surgical reversal. Techniques of reversal include unclipping and nerve grafting. Surgical clips can be used instead of surgical, thermal or ultrasonic ablation with the theoretic advantage of allowing reversal if the patient develops intolerable compensatory sweating. However, because permanent and irreversible perineural damage may occur to a nerve following the application of a clip, removal may not always result in return of sympathetic tone to the preoperative state.[2,44,45] In a 2009 study of thoracoscopic clipping for hyperhidrosis, 4.7% of the participants later underwent a reversal procedure for the development of CH. Of these patients, 48% reported a significant decrease of CH and 42% reported that the sweating at their original problem site remained controlled.[45] 68% of patients having a reversal within 6 months of the initial procedure reported substantial decrease in CH, versus 37% reporting substantial decrease in CH with a reversal procedure at greater than 6 months.[45]

SUMMARY

ETS is an effective surgical treatment for palmar, axillary, palmoplantar, and craniofacial hyperhidrosis, with reproducible improvement in more than 94% of patients.[2] Although initial immediate satisfaction rates are very high, patient satisfaction may decrease over time. This is mainly because of compensatory sweating, which occurs in many patients and can be a significant and bothersome problem that can decrease quality of life. Although surgical technique may reduce incidence of compensatory sweating and other side effects, patient characteristics such as anatomic location of sweating, age, body mass index, symptomatology, and comorbid conditions must also be taken into account. Selection of ideal surgical candidates using these parameters is key to the success of the surgery.[2] Patients must be made aware of not only the perioperative risks and benefits but also the long-term risks and benefits of this procedure.

REFERENCES

1. Hashmonai M, Kopelman D. History of sympathetic surgery. Clin Auton Res 2003;13(1):I6–9.

2. Cerfolio RJ, Milanez de Campos JR, Bryant AS, et al. The society of thoracic surgeons expert consensus for the surgical treatment of hyperhidrosis. Ann Thorac Surg 2011;91:1642–8.

3. Licht PB, Pilegaard HK. Severity of compensatory sweating after thoracoscopic sympathectomy. Ann Thorac Surg 2004;78:427–31.

4. Atkinson JL, Fode-Thomas NC, Fealey RD, et al. Endoscopic transthoracic limited sympathectomy for palmar-plantar hyperhidrosis: outcomes and complications during a 10-year period. Mayo Clin Proc 2011;86(8):721–9.

5. Marhold F, Izay B, Zacherl J, et al. Thoracoscopic and anatomic landmarks of Kuntz's nerve: implications for sympathetic surgery. Ann Thorac Surg 2008;86:1653–8.

6. Moran KT, Brady MP. Surgical management of primary hyperhidrosis. Br J Surg 1991;78:279–83.

7. Haxton HA. The sympathetic nerve supply of the upper limb in relation to sympathectomy. Ann R Coll Surg Engl 1954;14(4):247–66.

8. McCormack AC, Jarral OA, Shipolini AR, et al. Does the nerve of Kuntz exist? Interact Cardiovasc Thorac Surg 2011;13:175–8.

9. Walling HW, Swick BL. Treatment options for hyperhidrosis. Am J Clin Dermatol 2011;12(5):285–95.

10. Pather N, Partab P, Singh B, et al. Cervico-thoracic ganglion: its clinical implications. Clin Anat 2006; 19:323–6.

11. Glaser DA, Herbert AA, Pariser DM, et al. Facial Hyperhidrosis: best practice recommendations and special considerations. Cutis 2007;79(5): 29–32.

12. Reisfeld R, Pasternack GA, Daniels PD, et al. Severe plantar hyperhidrosis: an effective surgical solution. Am Surg 2013;79(9):845–53.

13. Oncel M, Sunam GS, Erdem E, et al. Bilateral thoracoscopic sympathectomy for primary hyperhidrosis: a review of 335 cases. Cardiovasc J South Af 2013; 24(4):137–40.

14. Liu Y, Yang J, Liu J, et al. Surgical treatment of primary palmar hyperhidrosis: a prospective randomized study comparing T3 and T4 sympathicotomy. Eur J Cardio Thorac Surg 2009;35:398–402.

15. Doolabh N, Horswell S, Williams M, et al. Thoracoscopic sympathectomy for hyperhidrosis: indications and results. Ann Thorac Surg 2004;77: 410–4.

16. Reisfeld R, Nguyen R, Pnini A. Endoscopic thoracic sympathectomy for hyperhidrosis. Experience with both cauterization and clamping methods. Surg Laparosc Endosc Percutan Tech 2002;12(4):255–67.

17. Miller DL, Bryant AS, Force SD, et al. Effect of sympathectomy level on incidence of compensatory hyperhidrosis after sympathectomy for palmar hyperhidrosis. J Thorac Cardiovasc Surg 2009; 138(3):581–5.

18. Yanagihara TK, Ibrahimiye A, Harris C, et al. Analysis of clamping versus cutting of T3 sympathetic nerve for severe palmar hyperhidrosis. J Thorac Cardiovasc Surg 2010;140(5):984–9.

19. Zhu LH, Chen L, Yang S, et al. Embryonic NOTES thoracic sympathectomy for palmar hyperhidrosis: results of a novel technique and comparison with the conventional VATS procedure. Surg Endosc 2013;11:4124–9.

20. Rua JF, Jatene FB, Milanez JR, et al. Robotic versus human camera holding in video-assisted thoracic sympathectomy: a single blind randomized trial of efficacy and safety. Interact Cardiovasc Thorac Surg 2009;8:195–9.

21. Hashimonai M, Kopelman D, Kein O, et al. Upper thoracic sympathectomy for primary palmar hyperhidrosis: long-term follow-up. Br J Surg 1992;79:268–71.

22. Dumont P, Denoyer A, Robin P. Long-term results of thoracoscopic sympathectomy for hyperhidrosis. Ann Thorac Surg 2004;78(5):1801–7.

23. Herbst F, Plas EG, Fugger R, et al. Endoscopic thoracic sympathectomy for primary hyperhidrosis of the upper limbs. A critical analysis and long-term results of 480 operations. Ann Surg 1994;220(1):86–90.

24. Drott C, Gothberg G, Claes G. Endoscopic transthoracic sympathectomy: an efficient and safe method for the treatment of hyperhidrosis. J Am Acad Dermatol 1995;33(1):78–81.

25. Askari A, Kordzadeh A, Lee GH, et al. Endoscopic thoracic sympathectomy for primary hyperhidrosis: a 16-year follow up in a single UK centre. Surgeon 2013;11:130–3.

26. Wolosker N, Munia MA, Kauffman P, et al. Is gender a predictive factor for satisfaction among patients undergoing sympathectomy to treat palmar hyperhidrosis? Clinics (Sao Paulo) 2010;65(6):583–6.

27. Deng B, Tan QY, Jiang YG, et al. Optimization of sympathectomy to treat palmar hyperhidrosis: the systematic review and meta-analysis of studies published during the past decade. Surg Endosc 2011;25(6):1893–901.

28. Neumayer C, Zacherl J, Holak G, et al. Limited endoscopic thoracic sympathetic block for hyperhidrosis of the upper limb: reduction of compensatory sweating by clipping T4. Surg Endosc 2004;18(1):152–6.

29. Baumgartner FJ, Reyes M, Sarkisyan GG, et al. Thoracoscopic sympathicotomy for disabling palmar hyperhidrosis: a prospective randomized comparison between two levels. Ann Thorac Surg 2011;92:2015–9.

30. Gossot D, Galetta D, Pascal A, et al. Long-term results for endoscopic thoracic sympathectomy for upper limb hyperhidrosis. Ann Thorac Surg 2003;75:1075–9.

31. Neumayer C, Panhofer P, Zacherl J, et al. Effect of endoscopic thoracic sympathetic block on plantar hyperhidrosis. Arch Surg 2005;140(7):676–80.

32. Licht PB, Ladegaard L, Pilegaard HK. Thoracoscopic sympathectomy for isolated facial blushing. Ann Thorac Surg 2006;81:1863–6.

33. Smidfelt K, Drott C. Late results of endoscopic thoracic sympathectomy for hyperhidrosis and facial blushing. Br J Surg 2011;98:1719–24.

34. Chiou TS. Chronological changes of postsympathectomy compensatory hyperhidrosis and recurrent sweating in patients with palmar hyperhidrosis. J Neurosurg Spine 2005;2:151–4.

35. Sihoe AD, Liu RW, Lee AK, et al. Is previous thoracic sympathectomy a risk factor for exertional heat stroke? Ann Thorac Surg 2007;84:1025–7.

36. Lai CL, Chen WJ, Liu YB, et al. Bradycardia and permanent pacing after bilateral thoracoscopic T2-sympathectomy for primary hyperhidrosis. Pacing Clin Electrophysiol 2001;24(4pt1):524–5.

37. Lin TS, Wang NP, Huang LC. Pitfalls and complication avoidance associated with transthoracic endoscopic sympathectomy for primary hyperhidrosis (analysis of 2200 cases). Int J Surg Investig 2001;2(5):377–85.

38. Ojimba TA, Cameron AE. Drawbacks of endoscopic thoracic sympathectomy. Br J Surg 2004;91(3):264–9.

39. de Andrade Filho LO, Kuzniec S, Wolosker N, et al. Technical difficulties and complications of sympathectomy in the treatment of hyperhidrosis: an analysis of 1731 cases. Ann Vasc Surg 2013;27(4):447–53.

40. Ribas Milanez de Campos J, Kauffman P, de Campos Werebe E, et al. Quality of life, before and after thoracic sympathectomy: report on 378 operated patients. Ann Thorac Surg 2003;76:886–91.

41. Weksler B, Blaine G, Souza ZB, et al. Transection of more than one sympathetic chain ganglion for hyperhidrosis increases the severity of compensatory hyperhidrosis and decreases patient satisfaction. J Surg Res 2009;156:110–5.

42. Wolosker N, Milanes de Campos JR, Kauffman P, et al. Evaluation of quality of life over time among 453 patients with hyperhidrosis submitted to endoscopic thoracic sympathectomy. J Vasc Surg 2012;55:154–6.

43. Milanez de Campos JR, Kauffman P, Wolosker N, et al. Axillary hyperhidrosis:T3/T4 versus T4 thoracic sympathectomy in a series of 276 cases. J Laparoendosc Adv Surg Tech 2006;16:598–603.

44. Latif MJ, Afthinos JN, Connery CP, et al. Robotic intercostal nerve graft for reversal of thoracic sympathectomy: a large animal feasibility model. Int J Med Robot 2008;4:258–62.

45. Sugimura H, Spratt EH, Compeau CG, et al. Thoracoscopic sympathetic clipping for hyperhidrosis: long-term results and reversibility. J Thorac Cardiovasc Surg 2009;137(6):1370–8.

Managing Hyperhidrosis
Emerging Therapies

Dee Anna Glaser, MD*, Timur A. Galperin, DO

KEYWORDS

- Hyperhidrosis • Topical botulinum toxin • Topical anticholinergics • Lasers • Ultrasound
- Radiofrequency

KEY POINTS

- Topical botulinum toxin A can be delivered through intact skin.
- Topical anticholinergic agents may provide efficacy with decreased adverse effects.
- Devices delivering energy such as lasers, ultrasound, and radiofrequency may reduce focal sweat.
- Limited data are available, and more research is needed.

INTRODUCTION

Treatment of severe axillary hyperhidrosis (HH) is limited to a few approved options. Botulinum toxin-A (BTX-A) injections provide temporary, albeit effective reduction in axillary sweating. Several surgical techniques have been used effectively for many years, but the invasiveness, down time, and adverse effects of such procedures are not ideal. Recently, the US Food and Drug Administration (FDA) approved a noninvasive microwave thermolysis device for axillary hyperhidrosis, which has shown long-term efficacy with minimal down time or adverse effects.[1,2] Additionally, there is a real need for therapies targeting nonaxillary HH and secondary forms of HH such as those related to antidepressant medications and menopause. As newer technologies are developed and older technologies refined, there is a potential to develop more effective treatment options for HH.

Botulinum Toxins

Topical botulinum toxin

Although onabotulinum toxin-A (onaBoNT-A) is FDA-approved for the treatment of axillary HH, it has been used effectively and safely to treat numerous hyperhidrotic areas. Multiple, repeat injections can be uncomfortable for some patients, especially in sensitive areas, such as the palms and soles. For these reasons, topical formulations of BTX-A are being developed and tested. A barrier to topical preparations is the large size of the botulinum toxin molecule. Revance Therapeutics, Incorporated (Newark, California), has developed a proprietary transport peptide that can be noncovalently coupled with the neurotoxin and successfully transport it across intact skin. A single, randomized, vehicle-controlled, within-patient comparison trial has been published with BTX-A (Botox, Allergan, Incorporated Irvine, California), 200 units in a proprietary vehicle delivery system in 12 patients.[3] The BTX-A solution and control vehicle were mixed with Cetaphil (Galderma, Fort Worth, TX) cream and applied once to the respective axillae for 60 minutes. Gravimetrically measured sweat reduction at 4 weeks after treatment was 65%, compared with 25.3% in the vehicle-treated axilla.[3] The 40% reduction in the quantitative sweat measurements was statistically significant ($P<.05$) There were no systemic adverse events, and no adverse events were considered to

Disclosure: D.A. Glaser has served as advisor for Allergan, Galderma, Miramar Labs, and Unilever. She has been an investigator and received research grants from Allergan, Miramar Labs, and Ulthera. T.A. Galperin has nothing to disclose.
Department of Dermatology, Saint Louis University School of Medicine, 1402 South Grand Boulevard-ABI, St Louis, MO 63104, USA
* Corresponding author.
E-mail address: glasermd@slu.edu

Dermatol Clin 32 (2014) 549–553
http://dx.doi.org/10.1016/j.det.2014.06.003
0733-8635/14/$ – see front matter © 2014 Elsevier Inc. All rights reserved.

be related to the BTX-A treatment. Mild folliculitis, erythema, eczema, and tenderness were noted locally; all of these were seen in the vehicle-only axilla.[3] Due to the small number of subjects, and short follow-up, long-term efficacy studies are warranted before topical BTX-A therapy can be accepted as an effective therapy for HH. Hopefully other body areas will be studied as well.

Topical Anticholinergics

Glycopyrrolate

First-line treatment for focal hyperhidrosis typically involves the use of aluminum chloride formulations, but their use has limited efficacy and is often irritating.[4] There is a real need to find a less irritating topical alternative, and several anticholinergics are being investigated. It is unknown whether benefit is a result of a focal effect on the eccrine duct (such as a physical block or chemical alteration) or on the gland only, or possibly both.

Like other anticholinergic medications, glycopyrrolate inhibits the acetylcholine-induced activation of sweat glands. To avoid the systemic anticholinergic adverse effects, topical formulations (0.5% to 4% cream, gel, solution, or pads) of glycopyrrolate have the potential to treat several different types of hyperhidrosis and several different body areas. Few case reports[5,6] and even fewer, randomized, placebo-controlled trials have looked at the effectiveness and safety of topical anitholinergic preperations on hyperhidrosis. Most of these studies evaluated gustatory hyperhidrosis, with limited data on other focal areas of hyperhidrosis.

A randomized, double-blind, placebo-controlled, crossover study of 13 diabetic patients with gustatory sweating showed that a 2-week application of 0.5% glycopyrrolate cream reduced sweating by 82%, as measured by sweat challenge testing.[7] A more recent study of 25 patients with craniofacial and gustatory hyperhidrosis showed that a single application of a 2% topical glycopyrrolate pad decreased sweat production by a mean of 61.8%, as measured by gravimetrics.[8] Although the results are promising, these studies evaluated a small subset of patients for a short period of time, which is not adequate to establish long-term safety or efficacy.

In a recent uncontrolled study of 35 patients with axillary hyperhidrosis, 1% glycopyrrolate cream was used once nightly for 4 weeks.[4] Only 9 of the 35 patients had a significant reduction in their sweating, based on a greater than 50% reduction in the patients' Dermatology Life Quality Index (DLQI) score.[4] However, the preparation was well tolerated without significant irritation or other compliance-limiting factors; 1 patient did develop

significant xerostomia and mydriasis. It is possible that the 1% concentration of the active drug or the formulation was not sufficient for the therapy to be effective.

In general, topical glycopyrrolate is well tolerated, with few reported adverse effects. These include headache, mydriasis, dry mouth, sore throat, skin irritation, and difficulty with accommodation.[4,7–10] Because of the reported effectiveness and safety of topical glycopyrrolate, larger randomized, placebo-controlled trials are necessary to establish the safety and efficacy of this therapy.

Oxybutynin

Oxybutynin, a competitive muscarinic receptor antagonist like other anticholinergic agents, has been used off-label for patients with hyperhidrosis. A new topical formulation of oxybutynin 3% topical gel was developed recently to increase tolerability of treatment compared with other transdermal formulations.[11] Adverse effects of topical oxybutynin gel are comparable to topical glycopyrrolate. These include skin irritation, dry mouth, constipation, headache, application site pruritus, nasopharyngitis, and dizziness.[11] Studies evaluating the safety and efficacy of topical oxybutynin gel for focal hyperhidrosis are warranted, because few effective topical therapies exist for hyperhidrosis.

Devices to Reduce Sweating

Devices that can deliver heat targeted at the eccrine units or to the surrounding tissue may be able to focally reduce sweat production via injury to the sweat gland. Devices currently exist that use various technologies such as laser, radiofrequency, and ultrasound to deliver energy to the soft tissue of skin. Some are applied externally to the skin, while others need to be inserted into the soft tissue. There are limited data on the use of these devices in treating HH, but they may hold promise. One device, MiraDry (Miramar Labs, Sunnyvale, California) uses microwave technology and is already cleared by the FDA to treat axillary HH; it is discussed in the article "Local Procedural Approaches for Axillary Hyperhidrosis" by Drs Glaser and Galperin in this issue.

Fractional microneedle radiofrequency treatment

Fractional microneedle radiofrequency (FMR) is a recently developed, minimally invasive procedure that delivers thermal energy to the reticular dermis, via rapid penetration with insulated microneedles, without causing epidermal injury. Bipolar radiofrequency energy is delivered in a fractional mode by 49 insulated microneedle electrodes (occupying a 1 cm^2 area) within the tip of a nonconductive probe. The bipolar electrode pins form a closed circuit with the treated skin, and can penetrate 0.5 to 3.5 mm below the skin surface.[12] Depending on the program selected, FMR can deliver up to 20 J of energy within 0.01 to 1 second, with a 5% or 10% coverage rate. In relation to the radiofrequency treatment level (range 1–20), and conduction time (range 10–1000 ms), the adjustable voltage can reach a maximum of 50 V.[12] FMR devices have been used effectively in the treatment of acne scars, facial pores, and wrinkles.[12] A recent pilot trial wanted to test the effectiveness of FMR for axillary HH, and provided 2 FMR treatments at 4-week intervals to 20 patients.[12]

All subjects received tumescent anesthesia prior to treatment. All axillae were treated with a total of 6 passes, starting at a depth of 3.5 mm for 150 milliseconds and at an energy level of 25 V for the first 2 passes. The second 2 passes went to a depth of 3.0 mm, and the final 2 passes were at a depth of 2.5 mm, with the duration (150 ms) and energy level (25 V) remaining constant.[12] Visible target area petechiae were the preferred irradiation end point. Ice packs were applied during treatment and for 10 minutes after treatment, and a hydrocolloid dressing was applied at the end.[12]

The mean HDSS score decreased from 3.5 at baseline to 2.3 2 months after treatment, and 60% of patients reached an HDSS score of 1 or 2 2 months after treatment. Histologic data from 3 patients showed a decrease in the number and size of apocrine and eccrine sweat glands 1 month after the final treatment. In most patients, only minimal adverse effects were noted, including mild pain, swelling, and redness after treatment. Compensatory HH was noted in 2 patients, and 1 patient had temporary arm numbness.[12] The results of this pilot study are promising, and further studies are needed for this novel treatment technique.

Long-pulsed 800 nm diode laser

Bechara and colleagues[13] used a long-pulsed 800 nm diode laser to treat 21 patients with axillary HH. In this half-side controlled trial, 5 treatment cycles were performed at 4 week intervals, using an energy setting of 50 mJ/cm^2 and pulse duration of 30 milliseconds (1.6 Hz). Sweating was reduced, as measured by gravimetric assessment, from 89 mg/min and 78 mg/min at baseline to 48 mg/min and 65 mg/min 4 weeks after the last treatment in the treated and control axillae, respectively.[13] Histologic examination of skin biopsies before and after the laser treatment revealed no change in the number or size of apocrine or eccrine glands, and no damage to the glands was found. The only adverse effect noted was temporary axillary skin depigmentation in a single

patient. The results were not statistically significant, and the authors noted that a larger sample size is needed to identify a therapeutic effect.

1064-nm Nd-YAG laser

A subdermal 1064-nm neodymium-doped yttrium aluminium garnet (Nd-YAG) laser has been used successfully for bromhidrosis,[14] and has the potential for treating axillary HH. Seventeen patients were numbed with tumescent anesthesia with or without sedation, and at least 1 1 mm incisions is made within the axillary crease. A 300 μm fiber optic laser cable transported in an 18-guage epidural needle was inserted into the incision. The 100 millisecond pulsed laser (40 Hz and 15 mJ) was guided slowly against the dermis in a crisscross pattern. Treatment of both axillae took 30 minutes.[14] Patients were followed every 3 months for a period of 12 to 43 months.

According to the patient's global assessment (PGA), there was an excellent result in 70.6% of patients, and based on the physician's global assessment, 82.3% of patients had good or excellent results. There was 1 relapse out of 17 patients within 5 months of treatment. Adverse effects included temporary dysesthesia in all patients, edema, alopecia (47.1%), and seroma formation (5.9%).[14] The results of this pilot study have yet to be replicated, and further research is needed to verify the efficacy of this technique.

A recent randomized, within-patient, case-controlled pilot study of 6 patients used a 1064-nm Nd-YAG laser externally at hair reduction settings to treat axillary HH.[15] Up to 6 laser hair reduction treatments were performed at 1-month intervals with 24 to 56 J/cm^2 (20 ms pulse duration) depending on the patient's skin type. Three subjects were followed for 1 month after the last treatment; 2 subjects were followed for 3 months, and 1 patient was followed for 13 months after the last treatment.

All of the patients reported good-to-excellent results 1 month after treatment, and 2 of 3 patients reported similar results 3 months after treatment, according to the PGA. There was decreased sweating in all 6 patients as noted by pre- and post-treatment starch iodine testing. There was no change in the sweat gland density or morphology on histologic analysis of the pre- and post-treatment biopsy samples.[15] The histologic findings suggest that sweat reduction is only temporary.

Ultrasound

The VASER (Solta Medical, Incorporated, Hayward, California) ultrasound system has been cleared by the FDA for body contouring and soft tissue emulsification. It focuses ultrasonic energy at the tip of a probe that is inserted into the soft tissue. Thirteen patients with axillary HH and/or bromihidrosis were treated with the system.[16] Local anesthesia and tumescent anesthesia were used in addition to intravenous sedation. A single 0.5 cm incision was made in the axillary crease; a protective skin port was sewn into the incision site, and the VASER probe was used with an amplitude setting of 80% in continuous mode during phase 1. The probe was passed evenly with radial strokes. Then the amplitude was reduced to 70%, and in continuous mode, phase 2 was completed. Lastly, an aspiration cannula was used to remove liquefied tissue and fluids. Based on 6-month post-treatment subjective scores, there was a mean 2.8 point reduction (on a scale of 1–5) in axillary sweating, and a mean 3 point improvement (on a scale of 1–5) in patient satisfaction. Only minor and temporary adverse effects were noted. A single case of blister formation, seroma formation, and hyperpigmentation was noted. All patients experienced temporary (1–2 days) postoperative pain. This study has promising results. Long-term follow-up and an objective assessment would have been beneficial in evaluating long-term efficacy. Further research is needed with this modality.

Externally applied ultrasound

Intense focused ultrasound (IFUS) has recently been developed to provide direct transcutaneous heat to the dermis and subcutaneous tissue for collagen remodeling. Ulthera (Ulthera, Incorporated, Mesa, Arizona) developed an IFUS device that has been cleared by the FDA and used for skin tightening and lifting procedures.[17] It has been tested for treating axillary HH (clinical trials.gov [NCT01708551, NCT01713673, NCT01713959 and NCT01722461]). The Ulthera system consists of a central power unit and monitor, a hand piece, and several interchangeable transducers, which vary in their energy level and depth of penetration. Energy levels vary from 0.5 to 10 J, with a frequency of 4 to 7 MHz, and pulse duration of 50 to 200 milliseconds. The hand piece uses diagnostic ultrasonography that is capable of imaging the epidermis/dermis, subcutaneous tissue, and blood vessels, and also contains the transducer for energy delivery.[17] The focused energy is absorbed by local dermal/subcutaneous tissues, leading to heat production and thermal injury. Thermal injury leads to wound healing and collagen remodeling. The heat may induce injury to the eccrine units, inducing a reduction in sweating.

Prior to the procedure, an anesthetic should be used to help with treatment discomfort. There is no particular anesthetic recommendation, but practitioners have used topical and local anesthetics, oral or intravenous analgesics, and conscious sedation, depending on the type and location of treatment. For cosmetic purposes, treatments are performed at 2 depths, with a single pass for each desired depth level. There is no specific aftercare for this procedure, and there is no down time after treatment. Temporary erythema and edema are common sequelae of treatment. Temporary numbness in the treatment area has also been reported.

At the time of writing, there are no publications outlining the results of the IFUS for HH, but the technology is promising.

SUMMARY

There is still a need for new therapies for the treatment of primary and secondary forms of hyperhidrosis. Understanding the location of the sweat glands and the pharmacology of sweat will help to drive new developments.

REFERENCES

1. Jacob C. Treatment of hyperhidrosis with microwave technology. Semin Cutan Med Surg 2013;32(1):2–8.
2. Glaser DA, Coleman WP, Fan LK, et al. A randomized, blinded clinical evaluation of a novel microwave device for treating axillary hyperhidrosis: the dermatologic reduction in underarm perspiration study. Dermatol Surg 2012;38(2):185–91. http://dx.doi.org/10.1111/j.1524-4725.2011.02250.x.
3. Glogau RG. Topically applied botulinum toxin type A for the treatment of primary axillary hyperhidrosis: results of a randomized, blinded, vehicle-controlled study. Dermatol Surg 2007;33(1 Spec No):S76–80. http://dx.doi.org/10.1111/j.1524-4725.2006.32335.x.
4. MacKenzie A, Burns C, Kavanagh G. Topical glycopyrrolate for axillary hyperhidrosis. Br J Dermatol 2013; 169(2):483–4. http://dx.doi.org/10.1111/bjd.12320.
5. Luh JY, Blackwell TA. Craniofacial hyperhidrosis successfully treated with topical glycopyrrolate. South Med J 2002;95(7):756–8.
6. Garnacho Saucedo GM, Moreno Jiménez JC, Jiménez Puya R, et al. Therapeutic hotline: topical glycopyrrolate: a successful treatment for craniofacial hyperhidrosis and eccrine hidrocystomas. Dermatol Ther 2010;23(1):94–7. http://dx.doi.org/10.1111/j.1529-8019.2009.01296.x.
7. Shaw JE, Abbott CA, Tindle K, et al. A randomised controlled trial of topical glycopyrrolate, the first specific treatment for diabetic gustatory sweating. Diabetologia 1997;40(3):299–301. http://dx.doi.org/10.1007/s001250050677.
8. Kim WO, Kil HK, Yoon KB, et al. Topical glycopyrrolate for patients with facial hyperhidrosis. Br J Dermatol 2008;158(5):1094–7. http://dx.doi.org/10.1111/j.1365-2133.2008.08476.x.

9. Kim WO, Kil HK, Yoon DM, et al. Treatment of compensatory gustatory hyperhidrosis with topical glycopyrrolate. Yonsei Med J 2003;44(4):579–82.
10. Cladellas E, Callejas MA, Grimalt R. A medical alternative to the treatment of compensatory sweating. Dermatol Ther 2008;21(5):406–8. http://dx.doi.org/10.1111/j.1529-8019.2008.00222.x.
11. Goldfischer ER, Sand PK, Thomas H, et al. Efficacy and safety of oxybutynin topical gel 3% in patients with urgency and/or mixed urinary incontinence: a randomized, double-blind, placebo-controlled study. Neurourol Urodyn 2013. http://dx.doi.org/10.1002/nau.22504.
12. Kim M, Shin JY, Lee J, et al. Efficacy of fractional microneedle radiofrequency device in the treatment of primary axillary hyperhidrosis: a pilot study. Dermatology 2013;227(3):243–9. http://dx.doi.org/10.1159/000354602.
13. Bechara FG, Georgas D, Sand M, et al. Effects of a long-pulsed 800-nm diode laser on axillary hyperhidrosis: a randomized controlled half-side comparison study. Dermatol Surg 2012;38(5):736–40. http://dx.doi.org/10.1111/j.1524-4725.2012.02339.x.
14. Goldman A, Wollina U. Subdermal Nd-YAG laser for axillary hyperhidrosis. Dermatol Surg 2008;34(6):756–62. http://dx.doi.org/10.1111/j.1524-4725.2008.34143.x.
15. Letada PR, Landers JT, Uebelhoer NS, et al. Treatment of focal axillary hyperhidrosis using a long-pulsed Nd:YAG 1064 nm laser at hair reduction settings. J Drugs Dermatol 2012;11(1):59–63.
16. Commons GW, Lim AF. Treatment of axillary hyperhidrosis/bromidrosis using VASER ultrasound. Aesthetic Plast Surg 2009;33(3):312–23. http://dx.doi.org/10.1007/s00266-008-9283-y.
17. Brobst RW, Ferguson M, Perkins SW. Ulthera: initial and six month results. Facial Plast Surg Clin North Am 2012;20(2):163–76, vi. http://dx.doi.org/10.1016/j.fsc.2012.02.003.

Resources for Hyperhidrosis Sufferers, Patients, and Health Care Providers

Lisa J. Pieretti, MBA

KEYWORDS

- Hyperhidrosis • Excessive sweating • Iontophoresis • Botox reimbursement
- Hyperhidrosis resources • Antiperspirants • Patient support • Patient advocacy

KEY POINTS

- Hyperhidrosis has a profoundly negative impact on sufferers' quality of life, yet medical professionals are scarcely trained in hyperhidrosis diagnosis and treatment.
- Sufferers do not seek treatment because they think nothing can be done, they do not know where to find medical care, or they are too embarrassed to discuss it with their physician.
- Bridging this gap is the International Hyperhidrosis Society (IHHS): a nonprofit organization that defines itself as the global authority in hyperhidrosis care and treatment, providing reliable information to the global, underserved community of sufferers and treatment providers.
- The Web site of the IHHS, www.SweatHelp.org, is the organization's virtual headquarters; content is translated into all languages, allowing the organization to truly serve an international audience.
- Medical professionals can discover more than 100 pages of resources through the IHHS from hyperhidrosis diagnosis and treatment to practice efficiency.

Founded in 2003 by an elite team of world-renowned physicians and experts in hyperhidrosis research, The International Hyperhidrosis Society (IHHS) has emerged as the global authority in hyperhidrosis care and treatment. Hyperhidrosis is a debilitating condition that causes the sufferer to sweat excessively, regardless of body temperature or external conditions. This nonprofit organization is committed to raising awareness and increasing the understanding and the quality of treatment of people who sweat excessively.

The IHHS is a distinctly 21st century organization; before its creation, there were few, if any, resources devoted to educating patients and health care providers on the cause and treatments of hyperhidrosis. The IHHS was created to address this gap in care because effective treatment of this disease can have a life-altering effect on a sufferer; likewise, for medical professionals, treating someone who has shouldered the burden and shame of hyperhidrosis can be extremely gratifying.

Hyperhidrosis is defined by copious uncontrollable sweating; it can affect any area of the body, but frequently occurs on the underarms, hands and/or feet, head, back, groin, chest, or other areas. Sweating excessively is physically uncomfortable; it can result in irritating or painful skin problems, such as bacterial or fungal overgrowth, infections, and maceration of the skin. It can also be an impediment to completing everyday tasks: someone with excessively sweating hands, for instance, can have great difficulty operating hand-held

Disclosure Statement: International Hyperhidrosis Society (IHHS) receives grants from Allergan, RA Fischer, and Procter & Gamble. The author has nothing to disclose.
International Hyperhidrosis Society, 2560 Township Road, Suite B, Quakertown, PA 18951, USA
E-mail address: LJP@SweatHelp.org

Dermatol Clin 32 (2014) 555–564
http://dx.doi.org/10.1016/j.det.2014.06.011
0733-8635/14/$ – see front matter © 2014 Elsevier Inc. All rights reserved.

derm.theclinics.com

devices, holding a steering wheel, and even holding a child.

The psychosocial and emotional damage that results from this condition can be devastating. Social anxiety and isolation due to the embarrassment and shame of sweating excessively leads to a limiting of ambitions and interactions with other people. Depression and decreased confidence are frequent side effects. Hyperhidrosis can also impose a financial burden: increased everyday expenses for necessities like extra clothing and antisweating supplies (not to mention the time it costs to manage the symptoms daily) add up over time. Some hyperhidrosis treatments are expensive, and obtaining insurance coverage for these, or any, hyperhidrosis treatment can be challenging.

The positive side of this condition is that outlook for patient care is continually improving, with credit going largely to the work of the IHHS. Effectively managing excessive sweating is possible: there is a range of treatment options available, based on both cutting-edge medical science and more traditional, but effective remedies. The one true obstacle to receiving care is the lack of knowledge in the medical community and the lack of information (and a preponderance of misinformation)

about hyperhidrosis among sufferers and their health care providers.

Over the past decade, the IHHS has begun removing this barrier to care through a major informational and educational outreach effort that targets both of these groups. SweatHelp.org is the IHHS's virtual global headquarters and central to much of this outreach; it provides users with a wealth of up-to-date and authoritative hyperhidrosis information and educational resources from world-renowned experts in the field.

SweatHelp.org receives more than 4000 visitors per day and is equipped with a dynamic translator tool that interprets content into every language (**Fig. 1**). The Web site includes a complete examination of all types of excessive sweating, from focal areas to night sweats, to compensatory, gustatory, and full-body sweating. All of the available treatment options are discussed as well as the pros and cons of each.

The Web site is divided into 4 sections, with content tailored to each particular audience: medical professional, hyperhidrosis sufferer, teen-aged or adolescent sufferer, and the media. The IHHS works diligently to ensure that the material on the Web site is the most reliable and current on the Internet.

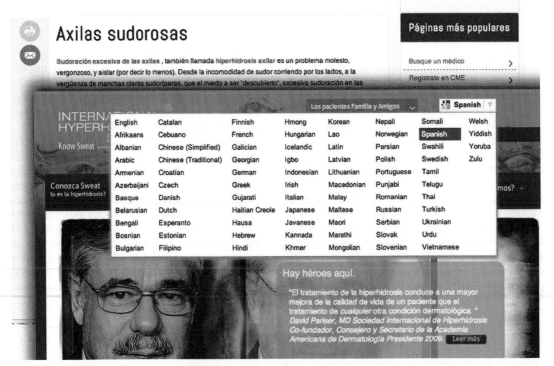

Fig. 1. SweatHelp.org receives more than 4000 visitors per day and is equipped with a dynamic translator tool that interprets content into every language. (*Courtesy of* International Hyperhidrosis Society, Quakertown, PA; with permission.)

There are many interactive materials for both patients and medical professionals, from the library of instructional training videos and modules (**Fig. 2**) demonstrating to medical professionals the nuanced administration of onabotulinumtoxinA injections to video testimonials clearly demonstrating the need for medical compassion and care.

Communicating with all segments of the hyperhidrosis community is important, but the experts

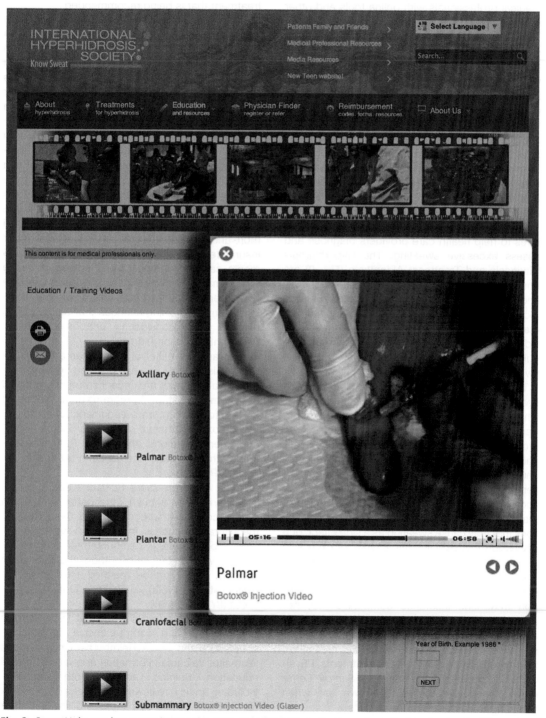

Fig. 2. SweatHelp.org has many interactive materials for both patients and medical professionals. (*Courtesy of* International Hyperhidrosis Society, Quakertown, PA; with permission.)

at the IHHS think that at the foundation of these improved-care opportunities are well trained and thoroughly knowledgeable medical professionals who treat, or are interested in treating, patients with excessive sweating. The IHHS, therefore, devotes a great deal of its resources to educating medical professionals with online tools and other in-person mentoring opportunities.

The SweatHelp.org section for medical professionals is vast. More than 100 pages of original, referenced content provide health care providers with an overview of how patients are affected by hyperhidrosis as well as its pathophysiology, epidemiology, and secondary causes. It also features complete analysis of treatment options presented in terms of areas affected, efficacy, adverse effects, treatment protocols, and long-term outcome. The Web site's library has an array of peer-reviewed articles and scientific literature available to all visitors who wish to review the research more deeply.

SweatHelp.org has many unique tools and features to help health care providers diagnose and assess excessive sweating. The Hyperhidrosis Diagnosis and Treatment Algorithms (Fig. 3) are one-of-a-kind tools that illustrate the diagnoses and all the possible courses of treatment of each focal area of excessive sweating (axillary, palmar, craniofacial, and so on) and provide treatment providers with clear, concise, and understandable guidelines for treating all types of excessive sweating.

These visual diagrams are very useful to both health care providers and their patients no matter where they are on their journey from diagnosis, to treatment, to successful management. Health care providers are also able to support patient understanding by requesting printed patient brochures from SweatHelp.org to distribute to their patients. Health care providers and sufferers can access helpful downloadable patient support materials, including a list of conditions and medications that may cause sweating as a side effect, or a discussion that explains the 2 types of excessive sweating (primary focal and secondary generalized).

All visitors to the site can make use of the range of insurance and reimbursement tools to help support treatment. Insurance companies may not routinely cover some treatments for hyperhidrosis and may require documentation of medical necessity when particular treatments are prescribed before deciding to pay for these treatments. Physicians can download and adapt the *Sample Letter of Medical Necessity* for their own use when providing documentation for patients.

This *Hyperhidrosis Preauthorization Request Form* may be downloaded and used to notify an insurance organization when a patient is diagnosed with hyperhidrosis and must demonstrate the degree to which their life is negatively affected by excessive sweating. There is also space on the form for a physician to note hyperhidrosis treatments that have already been tried and the next treatment that is being recommended.

Hyperhidrosis treatments have undergone major improvements in the 21st century. The 2004 US Food and Drug Administration approval of onabotulinumtoxinA injections for the treatment of axillary hyperhidrosis has helped to transform the lives of many thousands of sufferers and was a "game-changer" in the hyperhidrosis treatment regime. By "turning off" the process that leads to sweating excessively, the treatments allow sufferers to lead more normal lives, free, at least temporarily, from the overwhelming symptoms of hyperhidrosis.

However, as anyone who has pursued this line of therapy knows, treatments can be costly. Moreover, in this age of economic anxiety, when more and more people are carrying minimal health insurance, coming up with the money for treatments can seem impossible. Seeking coverage for treatment from insurance companies can likewise seem a daunting obstacle. There are, however, some promising avenues that sufferers can explore when considering onabotulinumtoxinA treatments for hyperhidrosis.

Allergan, the maker of Botox, has a Botox patient assistance program in place to help hyperhidrosis patients who are underinsured or uninsured get treatment. In fact, 3 programs offer a variety of options for patients who need financial help to pay for Botox treatments: Allergan's Botox Reimbursement Solutions, the Botox Patient Assistance Program, and the Botox Partnership for Access Program.

Botox Reimbursement Solutions (https://www.botoxreimbursement.us/) puts patients in touch with a counselor who can guide them through the insurance process, including answering questions about coverage, reimbursement policies, insurance verifications, prior authorizations, or claim appeals. They can be reached toll-free in the United States at (800) 44-BOTOX, Option 4 or via fax at (877) 530-6680.

Medical professionals who treat hyperhidrosis patients can find comprehensive support resources on the Botox Reimbursement Solutions Web site. Valuable information about on-site staff education, training, and in-depth support—including policy reviews and analysis of Botox reimbursement that can improve billing and coding and other office processes, which decrease the chances of having claims denied.

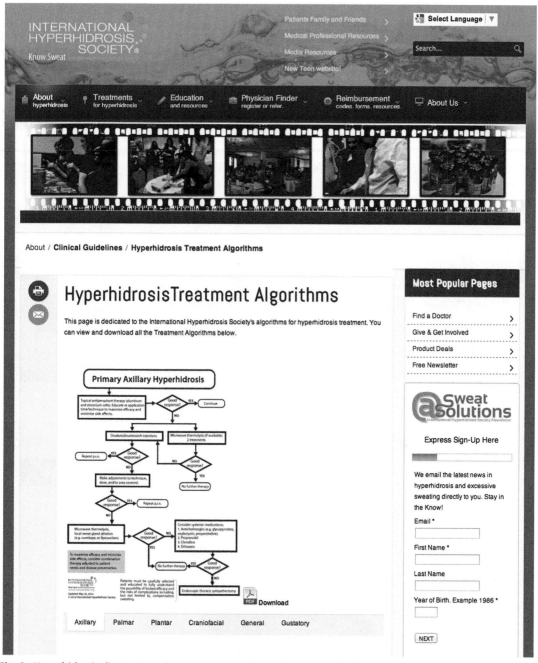

Fig. 3. Hyperhidrosis diagnosis and treatment algorithms. (*Courtesy of* International Hyperhidrosis Society, Quakertown, PA; with permission.)

For patients who do not have insurance or who are underinsured, Allergan's Botox Patient Assistance Program can help. Through this program, Allergan will donate Botox vials for the treatment of financially eligible patients. Patients can download the Botox Patient Assistance Program Application online. Call toll-free in the United States at (800) 44-BOTOX, Option 6 for help or more information.

The Botox Partnership for Access Program was created to help insured patients who struggle to meet their out-of-pocket Botox treatment costs. Patients who qualify will receive a debit card to be used for either future medical or personal expenses. The debit card can also be reused for future credits if the treating physician determines a need for re-treatment within 120 days of the first treatment. Patients can find out if they are eligible via the Botox Partnership for Access Web site and learn more about each of these incredibly helpful programs. Patients must be at least 18 years of age to participate.

Iontophoresis device maker, R.A. Fischer Company, also has an option to rent iontophoresis devices so people can try out their device before purchasing. This rental plan is especially useful for parents who are trying the device for children. It makes sense and is inexpensive. R.A. Fischer has excellent customer service, and those interested in purchasing or renting and even those with questions may contact Bill Schuler at (800) 525-3467. They are truly dedicated to patients and to ensure that they are using their machines properly. On request, they have walked patients through their initial

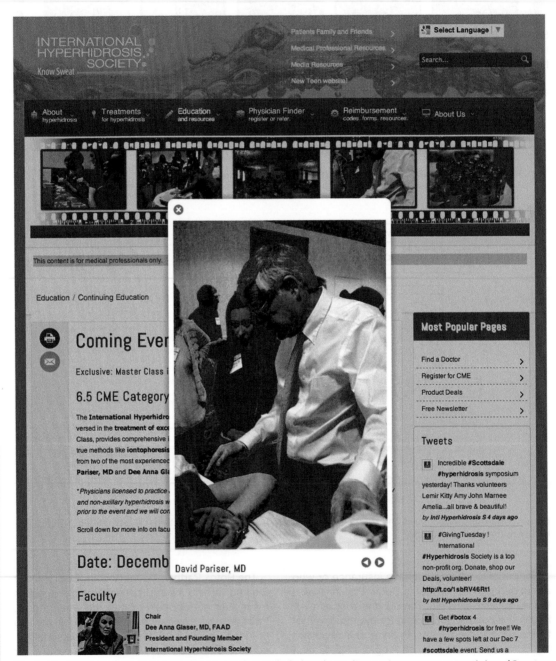

Fig. 4. The IHHS conducts 1-day, CME seminars that include hands-on, live-patient treatment training. (*Courtesy of* International Hyperhidrosis Society, Quakertown, PA; with permission.)

treatment setup and got them on their way with the treatment.

For both patients and dermatologists, Fischer offers a 45-day unconditional money-back guarantee. For patients, they also offer rental programs with affordable monthly terms and the option to buy. For dermatologists, the Fischer Company offers discounts for internal use devices as well as for devices dermatologists can resell to their patients.

The ever-popular topical antiperspirant, Secret Clinical Strength, has a loyalty program for its customer base: they can buy 4 Secret Clinical Strength products and send in the UPCs from the bottom of the box, and the brand will send the customer a coupon for 1 FREE Secret Clinical Strength deodorant/antiperspirant. Download the PDF and more information at http://www.secret.com/Loyalty-Program.aspx.

In addition to the Web site, several times a year the IHHS conducts 1-day, continuing medical education (CME) seminars (**Fig. 4**) that include hands-on, live-patient treatment training for medical professionals with some of the premiere experts in hyperhidrosis care in the world. These events offer comprehensive tutorials on the cause of hyperhidrosis and its quality-of-life implications. All aspects of care are examined—from guidelines for integrating hyperhidrosis care into a health care practice to live-patient treatment instruction on all body areas that exhibit excessive sweating. All

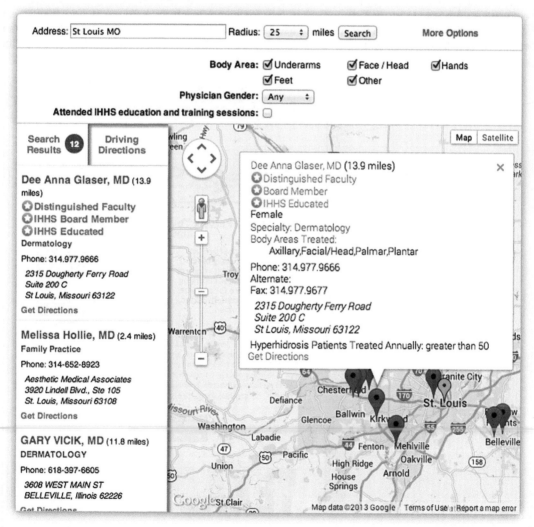

Fig. 5. Physician Finder is the organization's global registry of physicians and medical professionals who treat excessive sweating. (*Courtesy of* International Hyperhidrosis Society, Quakertown, PA; with permission.)

treatment methodologies, including Botox injections and iontophoresis administration, are demonstrated.

These seminars are extremely beneficial to the hyperhidrosis community because they help to spread knowledge and provide more opportunities to improve hyperhidrosis treatment outcomes. (A few fortunate hyperhidrosis patients also receive free expert treatment at these events.) After completing the class, all attendees are awarded special status in the *Physician Finder* database on SweatHelp.org.

Physician Finder (**Fig. 5**) is the organization's global registry of physicians and medical professionals who treat excessive sweating. It is available to all patients and health care providers, and those who participate in one of the IHHS's CME seminars receive special designation by their name, indicating their proficiency in hyperhidrosis treatment.

Communication and outreach are important aspects of the IHHS's philosophy, which helps connect a lively global community of patients, loved ones, and doctors who share the experience of living with and treating hyperhidrosis. Executive Director of the organization, Lisa Pieretti, strives to keep the hyperhidrosis community involved with the organization and encourages users to communicate with the IHHS community through its Contact Us page or through one of the many social media platforms, like Facebook and Twitter.

The IHHS has a free e-newsletter, *SweatSolutions* (**Fig. 6**), which has more than 42,000 subscribers and features stories that impact or relate to the evolving world of hyperhidrosis impact, research, and care.

Of particular importance and focus for the IHHS are children and teen hyperhidrosis sufferers. Hyperhidrosis age of onset is during childhood or adolescence and living with it during these early years can be heart-wrenching for both kids and parents. Reaching sufferers during these early years has been shown to be especially important and impactful. Addressing this need is the

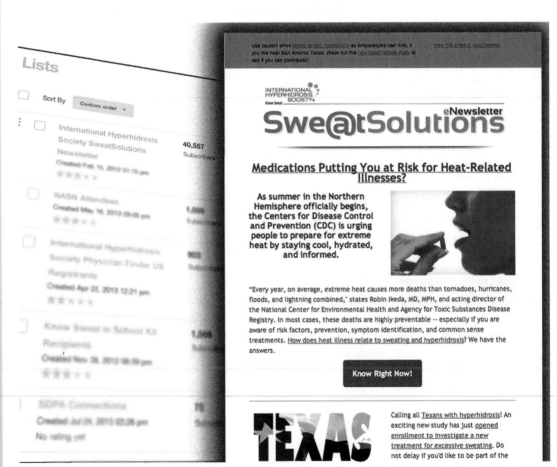

Fig. 6. The IHHS has a free e-newsletter, SweatSolutions, which has more than 42,000 subscribers and features stories that impact or relate to the evolving world of hyperhidrosis impact, research, and care. (*Courtesy of* International Hyperhidrosis Society, Quakertown, PA; with permission.)

dedicated Web site for adolescents www.Sweat Ometer.org (**Fig. 7**) Information in this section is delivered in a way that a tween or teen would find more relatable.

School nurses also play a role in the IHHS's educational outreach because they have a unique vantage and can sometimes become the most constant and trusted health care provider during a child's school-aged years. Teaching school nurses to recognize the symptoms of hyperhidrosis and providing them with knowledge and information to pass along to kids and their parents is a successful start to hyperhidrosis care. (Medical opinion is in agreement that the earlier excessive sweating is diagnosed and treated, the weaker the impact of hyperhidrosis on a sufferer's life.)

The IHHS's *Know Sweat in School* program provides kits that are specifically designed to support the school nurse in her outreach to kids (and their parents) who may be affected by excessive sweating. Thousands of kits have been distributed to school nurses across the US by specific request; they contain teen-focused visual aids, literature, and antisweat products.

SweatHelp.org has a Deals and Discounts section that provides discounted products favored by the excessive sweating community, which are typically lesser known among the general public. Products made exclusively for excessive sweating, like sweat-absorbent insoles for excessively sweating feet, are offered at an exclusive, discounted rate. Many of the items available on this page are manufactured by small business leaders who developed innovative ideas to manage their own excessive sweating. This theme of excessive sweaters helping out other excessive sweaters when they become adults is a repeated theme within the hyperhidrosis community and is another element of community interaction and participation that the IHHS and its Web site work hard to foster.

Another avenue of participation in the global hyperhidrosis community is to get involved in one of the various clinical and/or market research opportunities available through SweatHelp.org. Sufferers can participate in a long-term genetic research study being conducted by genetic experts at the Albert Einstein College of Medicine. Hyperhidrosis is a condition that is frequently shared across generations; this study is pioneering new ways of understanding and treating excessive sweating. Many members of the IHHS

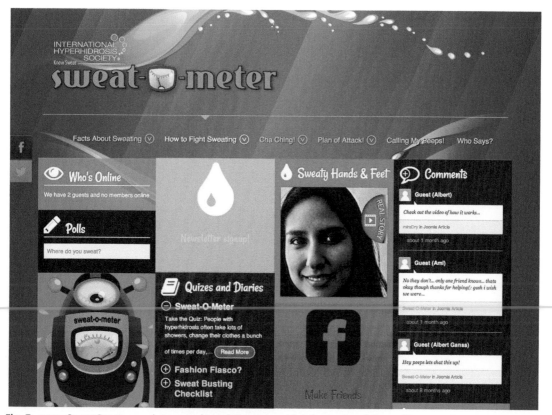

Fig. 7. www.SweatOmeter.org is targeted to adolescents, with information delivered in a way that a tween or teen would find more relatable. (*Courtesy of* International Hyperhidrosis Society, Quakertown, PA; with permission.)

community—along with many of their family members—have already participated and the findings may be significant to treatment development.

Finally, there is the content directed specifically to the media, which helps increase awareness about hyperhidrosis among the general public with things like checklists to help determine if sweating is excessive, how to survive a job interview with hyperhidrosis, and so much more. Overall, the IHHS offers a vast resource for improving the lives of people who suffer with and treat excessive sweating. The Web site emphasizes the importance of understanding the disease and the variety of treatment options available to treat all types of excessive sweating. It also stresses the powerful degree to which hyperhidrosis can affect a sufferer's life and the equally powerful impact that treating it can have on a patient as well as a health care provider.

Improving lives for patients with excessive sweating can be done effectively and with a variety of treatment methods, some very simple, some incredibly complex. What is required of either patient or health care provider is a modest investment of time to educate themselves, along with some patience and persistence to overcome some of the still-remaining obstacles to effective hyperhidrosis care. To support the entire process is the IHHS organization, with its noble mission, which inspired one of its founding board members, David Pariser, MD, to remark about caring for patients with excessive sweating: "Treating hyperhidrosis leads to a greater improvement of a patient's quality of life than treatment of *any* other dermatologic condition. Treating someone who suffers with excessive sweating can be a deeply rewarding experience."

Incorporating Diagnosis and Treatment of Hyperhidrosis into Clinical Practice

David M. Pariser, MD[a,b],*

KEYWORDS

- Primary focal hyperhidrosis • Medical necessity • Diagnosis • Reimbursement

KEY POINTS

- Treatments for hyperhidrosis lead to a great improvement in patient quality of life.
- Proper billing and coding are needed to document diagnosis and treatment and assure proper reimbursement.
- Providers may buy and bill botulinum toxin or prescribe it as a drug for any individual patient.
- Algorithms for treating various forms of hyperhidrosis can help clinicians decide on the best treatments.

Is hyperhidrosis a cosmetic condition for which patients should pay out of pocket for treatment or is it a true medical disease that should be considered necessary to treat and therefore covered by health insurance? How this question is answered by the provider will largely determine how treatments are incorporated into a busy clinical practice.

For providers who choose to treat hyperhidrosis as a cosmetic condition, the provider need not bother with insurance precertification, determination of medical necessity, or billing. Whether the patient is getting iontophoresis, botulinum toxin injections, local surgery, or treatment with a device such as the miraDry microwave system (Miramar Labs, Inc., Santa Clara, CA, USA), the provider simply collects a cash payment from the patient, often before the procedure is performed.

By considering hyperhidrosis a true disease that is medically necessary to treat, the financial barrier to care is lessened and far more people with the condition are able to receive treatment. Expensive treatments such as botulinum toxin injections or miraDry procedures are inaccessible for many patients if out-of-pocket payment is required. Some high-deductible health plans also present an obstacle to care if these deductibles have not been met already, which is often the case for an otherwise healthy young person with low health care expenses—the primary demographic of patients with hyperhidrosis. Curiously, the medical necessity of one of the most expensive and most invasive treatments, endoscopic thoracic sympathectomy, is seldom questioned by insurance payers and is usually covered.

If the full range of hyperhidrosis treatments is made available, including topical and systemic therapies, iontophoresis, botulinum toxin injections, miraDry microwave procedures, and local surgery, the provider should get to know the coverage policies of the major health plans in the local service area. Some plans will require a stepwise ladder of treatments; usually failure of or intolerance to topical and oral systemic therapies is required before other treatments, such as iontophoresis or botulinum toxin injections, will be considered for

a International Hyperhidrosis Society, Quakertown, PA 18951, USA; b Department of Dermatology, Eastern Virginia Medical School, 601 Medical Tower, Norfolk, VA 23507, USA
* Department of Dermatology, Eastern Virginia Medical School, 601 Medical Tower, Norfolk, VA 23507.
E-mail address: dpariser@pariserderm.com

Dermatol Clin 32 (2014) 565–574
http://dx.doi.org/10.1016/j.det.2014.06.010
0733-8635/14/$ – see front matter © 2014 Elsevier Inc. All rights reserved.

coverage. Treatment with the miraDry microwave device is uniformly not covered by insurance.

Contacting a medical director of the major health plans in a provider's local service area may be helpful to ascertain whether the health plan uses any particular criteria to determine medical necessity or follows guidelines for clinical decision making regarding coverage of treatments for hyperhidrosis. One example of an ill-conceived criterion of medical necessity is the requirement that a patient exhibit signs of maceration or infection before axillary hyperhidrosis is considered medically necessary to treat, when in fact maceration and infection are seldom seen in uncomplicated primary focal axillary hyperhidrosis. If a health plan does not have criteria for determining the medical necessity for treatment of hyperhidrosis, providers can offer to help develop them. Health plans pay attention to published literature, especially that which is peer-reviewed and presents good science. Published treatment algorithms, such as those developed by the International Hyperhidrosis Society (see **Figs. 2–7**), may be a helpful resource when developing a carrier's precertification process.

A letter of medical necessity is usually required to document the need for treatment of hyperhidrosis for any individual patient. Items that should be in this letter include the severity of the disorder, examples of professional or psychosocial disability or impairment, and a history of previous treatments. Severity may be documented on the Hyperhidrosis Disease Severity Scale (HDSS), a validated patient-reported metric that is used in most clinical trials of hyperhidrosis treatments. The HDSS is described in more detail in the article by Pariser and Ballard elsewhere in this issue. Documenting a specific incident of extreme embarrassment or an example when the disorder prevented or ruined a social or professional encounter can be compelling. If failure of a previous treatment is required before a patient can advance to a more expensive or invasive one, it is important to have reasonable periods for the "failed" treatments. For example, it is not reasonable to require failure of a topical or systemic treatment for a period of 6 months if the agent is clearly not producing a satisfactory result or is not being adequately tolerated.

BEST PRACTICES FOR PATIENT FLOW

When a patient calls for an appointment and excessive sweating is identified as the reason for the visit, the patient should be referred to a source of authoritative information, such as the International Hyperhidrosis Society Web site (sweathelp.

org). Office visits can be much more productive when patients become informed beforehand.

Providers should have an intake form that can be sent to the patient in advance or completed at the time of the visit to capture information such as past medical history relating to the sweating, HDSS score (described in the article by Pariser and Ballard elsewhere in this issue), and previous treatment history.

Nonphysician clinicians, such as nurse practitioners, physician assistants, and medical assistants, can be a great help in aspects of initial evaluation and diagnosis, formulating a treatment plan, prescribing topical and systemic agents, performing iontophoresis and microwave treatments, and administering botulinum toxin injections. The specific tasks assigned to the nonphysician clinicians should be commensurate with their licensure and conform to training and supervision requirements of state law and standard of medical care. Everyone on the care team can participate in patient education about the disease and its treatments.

Providers should use resources such as the International Hyperhidrosis Society Web which has physician and patient educational material as well as administrative support. Manufacturers of some of the drugs and devices used to treat hyperhidrosis also have patient and provider support material (see the article by Pieretti elsewhere in this issue).

BILLING AND CODING FOR HYPERHIDROSIS AND ITS TREATMENTS

Proper billing and coding for hyperhidrosis diagnosis and treatments will ensure that the condition is reported properly and the provider is appropriately reimbursed. Proper coding involves the use of an ICD-9 (*International Classification of Diseases, Ninth Revision*) code for the diagnosis, a CPT (*Current Procedural Terminology*) code for the procedure performed, and, if applicable, an HCPCS (Healthcare Common Procedure Coding System) drug code (commonly called a *J code*), which is used to identify injectable drugs such as botulinum toxin.

ICD-9 Codes

The ICD-9 codes are used to document the diagnosis. Most patients who have excessive sweating from one or more body sites and are diagnosed with primary focal hyperhidrosis are appropriately coded with the ICD-9 code 705.21. If there is a primary cause for the hyperhidrosis, such as a medication, endocrinopathy, or neurologic issue, the IDC-9 code for secondary hyperhidrosis is used, which is 705.22.

ICD-10 Codes

Scheduled to be implemented in October, 2015, after a year delay, diagnosis codes using ICD-10 will preplace ICD-9 in the United States. These codes will be more specific than the ICD-9 codes and will more properly describe the diagnosis (**Fig. 1**).

CPT Codes

Iontophoresis

The primary CPT code for iontophoresis treatments is 97033, which is defined as, "Iontophoresis, each 15 minutes." Depending on how many body areas are treated, usually more than one unit of 97033 will be billed. The standard treatment time for iontophoresis is usually 20 minutes to each body part, with the polarity of the current reversed after the first 10 minutes. Treatments to both hands, both feet, or one hand and one foot for 20 minutes generates 2 billing units of code 97033. Treatment of all 4 extremities should take 40 minutes of iontophoresis and would generate 3 billing units of 97033. If any separately identifiable service is also provided, such as a physician visit for evaluation of treatment progress, it is appropriate to also use a code for evaluation and management (E&M) services (CPT codes 99211–99213), depending on the intensity of the service rendered. In this case, when an E&M service is being provided on the same day as the iontophoresis, the modifier "−25" should be appended to the E&M code to indicate that it was a separately identifiable service.

Botulinum toxin injections

Two specific CPT codes are used for botulinum toxin injections, one for the axillae and one for the scalp, face, and/or neck. Injections into other areas on the extremities, including the hands and feet, are properly reported with CPT code 64999, which is defined as, "Unlisted procedure, nervous system." Use of the 64999 code usually requires manual processing and often requires written medical documentation. There is usually no predetermined value for the 64999 code. The code for axillary injections is 64650 and is properly used when one or both axillae are injected. CPT code 64653 applies to injections in any area on face, scalp, or neck, and only one unit of this code may be billed per day.

HCPCS J Codes

The J code J0585, "Injection, onabotulinumtoxinA, 1 unit," is used to report the physician-supplied botulinum toxin of the Botox brand, the only botulinum toxin approved by the US Food and Drug Administration (FDA) for the treatment of hyperhidrosis. The J0585 code only applies to *1 unit* of botulinum toxin. Because 100 units are usually used and for axillae and up to 300 units may be used at one treatment for other areas, such as hands and feet, it is important to bill with the appropriate number of billing units of the J code.

BILLING OPTIONS FOR BOTULINUM TOXIN TREATMENTS

Botulinum toxin injections may be provided to patients in 2 ways if the procedure and the cost of the drug will be covered by insurance. Either the practice can buy the drug and bill the patient's insurance ("buy-and-bill") or the botulinum toxin can be written as a prescription.

In the buy-and-bill model, the provider purchases the botulinum toxin and performs the injections, and bills both the CPT code for the injection services and the J code for the botulinum toxin. Usually a preauthorization process is required before the injections are administered to assure payment. Medical necessity will need to be documented, but different insurance payers will have

L74.5 Focal hyperhidrosis
  L74.51 Primary focal hyperhidrosis
    L74.510 ...... axilla
    L74.511 ...... face
    L74.512 ...... palms
    L74.513 ...... soles
    L74.519 ...... unspecified
  L74.52 Secondary focal hyperhidrosis
 L74.8 Other eccrine sweat disorders
 L74.9 Eccrine sweat disorder, unspecified

Fig. 1. ICD-10 codes for hyperhidrosis effective in October, 2015.

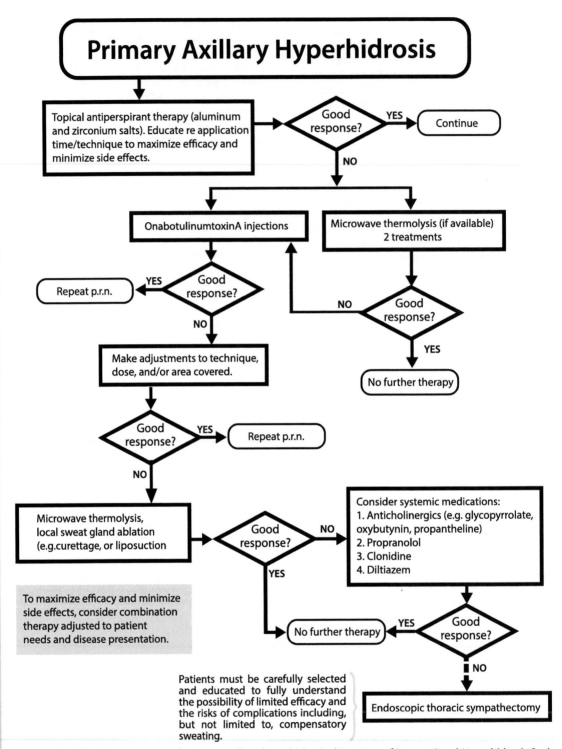

Fig. 2. Algorithm for treatment of primary axillary hyperhidrosis. (*Courtesy of* International Hyperhidrosis Society, Quakertown, PA; with permission.)

different rules about determination of medical necessity. Providers should become familiar with the preauthorization procedures of the various companies to ease the process. Providers should also be aware that preauthorization does not always guarantee payment. Treatments may be preauthorized as a covered service on the health plan, but the insurance carrier may determine

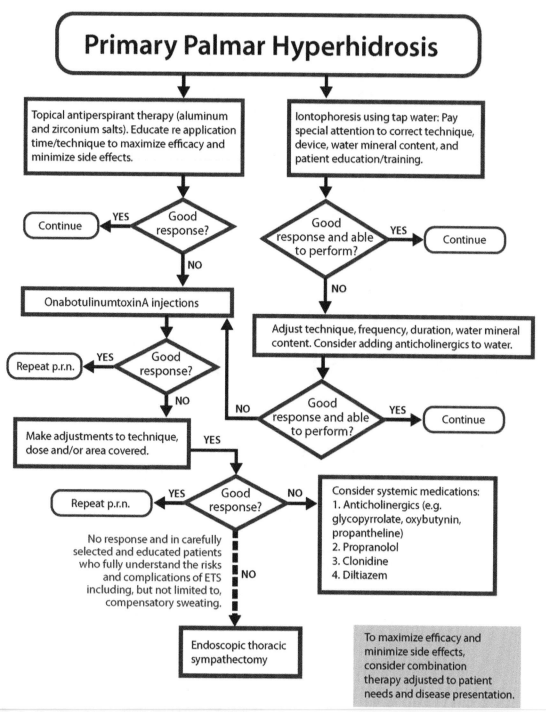

Fig. 3. Algorithm for treatment of primary palmar hyperhidrosis. (*Courtesy of* International Hyperhidrosis Society, Quakertown, PA; with permission.)

retrospectively that a particular treatment for a particular patient was not medically necessary. In this case, the provider may have to appeal the denial of a claim, and may eventually have to absorb the cost of the botulinum toxin, which is usually more than the physician service. Because botulinum toxin provided to the patient on the buy-and-bill method is considered a medical benefit (as opposed to a pharmacy benefit), the patient may have less of a copay, but that is highly

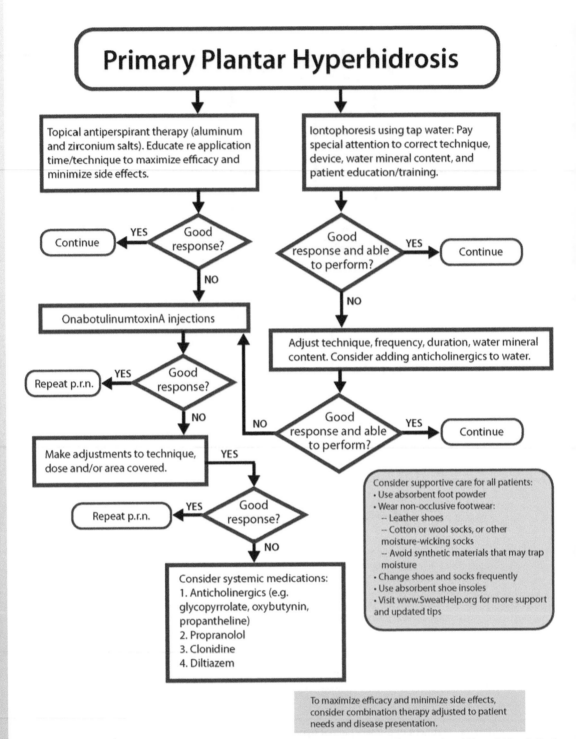

Fig. 4. Algorithm for treatment of primary plantar hyperhidrosis. (*Courtesy of* International Hyperhidrosis Society, Quakertown, PA; with permission.)

variable depending on the terms of a patient's individual health plan coverage.

The other billing option for the provider is to prescribe the botulinum toxin for the individual patient.

A written or electronic prescription is sent to the patient's pharmacy, which is often a mail-order specialty pharmacy directed by the health plan, but also could be a local retail pharmacy. In this case,

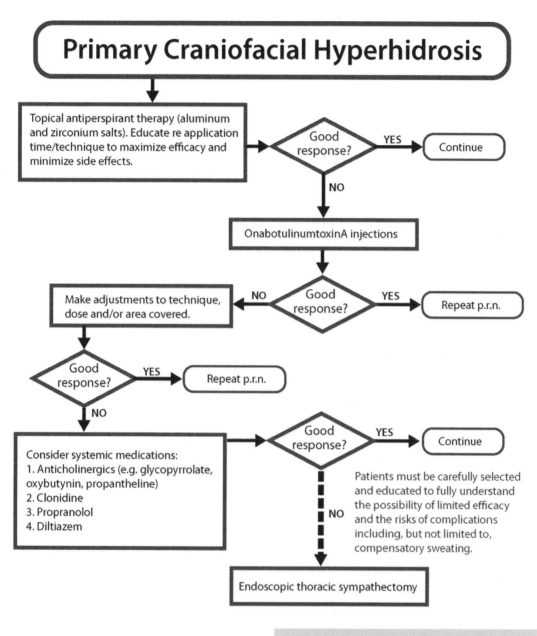

Fig. 5. Algorithm for treatment of primary craniofacial hyperhidrosis. (*Courtesy of* International Hyperhidrosis Society, Quakertown, PA; with permission.)

the pharmacy is responsible for obtaining the necessary preauthorization for the drug. The pharmacy then provides the botulinum toxin to the provider, who administers it in the office. The provider should still obtain preauthorization for the injection service, and should bill using the proper CPT code for the anatomic area being treated. This method of billing does not put the provider at risk for the cost of the botulinum toxin. The patient will be responsible for a copay for the drug, and for the injection service. The copay will vary according to the terms of the patient's individual policy.

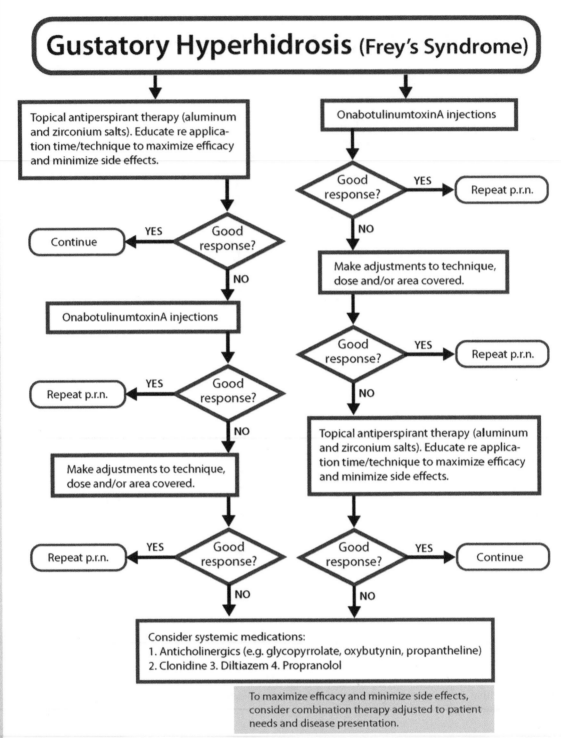

Fig. 6. Algorithm for treatment of gustatory hyperhidrosis (Frey syndrome). (*Courtesy of* International Hyperhidrosis Society, Quakertown, PA; with permission.)

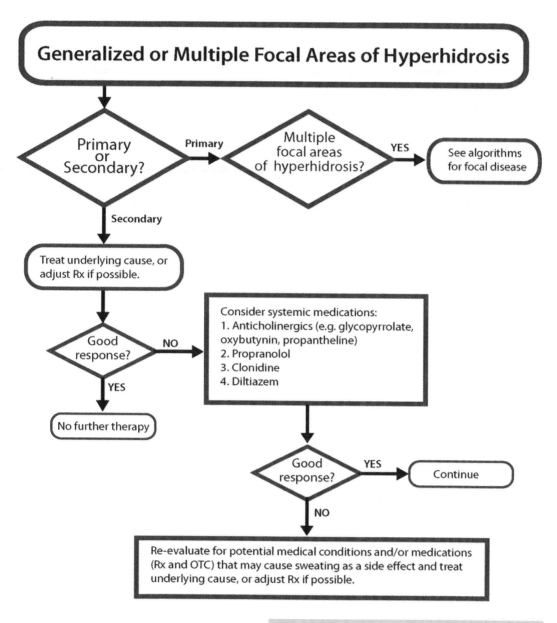

Fig. 7. Algorithm for treatment of generalized or multiple focal areas of hyperhidrosis. (*Courtesy of* International Hyperhidrosis Society, Quakertown, PA; with permission.)

BILLING FOR OTHER SERVICES RELATING TO HYPERHIDROSIS TREATMENTS

The starch-iodine test for determining the extent of excessive sweating in any particular area is described in the article by Trindade de Almieda elsewhere in this issue. No CPT code exists for this procedure, and usually no additional reimbursement is provided for this procedure. It is considered part of the service covered by CPT codes 64650 and 64653.

Local surgical procedures for the treatment of axillary hyperhidrosis, such as liposuction, subcutaneous curettage, and laser treatments, are also not described by any CPT code and are seldom reimbursed by insurance.

Similarly, although miraDry microwave treatments are approved by the FDA for axillary hyperhidrosis, they have no associated CPT code and are usually not covered by insurance. Some patients may try to obtain reimbursement on their own.

SUMMARY

Treatment of primary focal hyperhidrosis is easily learned and can greatly improve the quality of life of patients with this disease. Patients with successfully treated hyperhidrosis often become loyal and supportive spokespersons. Through the development of efficient office management procedures, the diagnosis and treatment of these patients can be easily integrated into office practice and be economically viable for a busy dermatologic practice. Properly trained and supervised nonphysician clinicians, such as nurse practitioners, physician assistants, and medical assistants, can greatly enhance efficiency through providing most of the treatments, patient education, and follow-up for hyperhidrosis, allowing physicians to concentrate on diagnosis and treatment planning.

To help providers with therapeutic decision making for patients with hyperhidrosis, the International Hyperhidrosis Society published algorithms for the various types of generalized and focal hyperhidrosis (**Figs. 2–7**). More information and practice aids are described in the article by Pieretti elsewhere in this issue, and can be found on the International Hyperhidrosis Society Web site (sweathelp.org).

Index

Dermatol Clin 32 (2014) 575–578
http://dx.doi.org/10.1016/S0733-8635(14)00090-4
0733-8635/14/$ – see front matter © 2014 Elsevier Inc. All rights reserved.

United States Postal Service

Statement of Ownership, Management, and Circulation
(All Periodicals Publications Except Requestor Publications)

1. Publication Title
Dermatologic Clinics

2. Publication Number
0 0 0 - 7 0 5

3. Filing Date
9/14/14

4. Issue Frequency
Jan, Apr, Jul, Oct

5. Number of Issues Published Annually
4

6. Annual Subscription Price
$365.00

7. Complete Mailing Address of Known Office of Publication (Not printer) (Street, city, county, state, and ZIP+4®)
Elsevier Inc.
360 Park Avenue South
New York, NY 10010-1710

Contact Person
Stephen R. Bushing

Telephone (Include area code)
215-239-3688

8. Complete Mailing Address of Headquarters or General Business Office of Publisher (Not printer)
Elsevier Inc., 360 Park Avenue South, New York, NY 10010-1710

9. Full Names and Complete Mailing Addresses of Publisher, Editor, and Managing Editor (Do not leave blank)

Publisher (Name and complete mailing address)
Linda Belfus, Elsevier Inc., 1600 John F. Kennedy Blvd., Suite 1800, Philadelphia, PA 19103-2899

Editor (Name and complete mailing address)
Joanne Husovski, Elsevier Inc., 1600 John F. Kennedy Blvd., Suite 1800, Philadelphia, PA 19103-2899

Managing Editor (Name and complete mailing address)
Adrianne Brigido, Elsevier Inc., 1600 John F. Kennedy Blvd., Suite 1800, Philadelphia, PA 19103-2899

10. Owner (Do not leave blank. If the publication is owned by a corporation, give the name and address of the corporation immediately followed by the names and addresses of all stockholders owning or holding 1 percent or more of the total amount of stock. If not owned by a corporation, give the names and addresses of the individual owners. If owned by a partnership or other unincorporated firm, give its name and address as well as those of each individual owner. If the publication is published by a nonprofit organization, give its name and address.)

Full Name	Complete Mailing Address
Wholly owned subsidiary of	1600 John F. Kennedy Blvd, Ste. 1800
Reed/Elsevier, US holdings	Philadelphia, PA 19103-2899

11. Known Bondholders, Mortgagees, and Other Security Holders Owning or Holding 1 Percent or More of Total Amount of Bonds, Mortgages, or Other Securities. If none, check box ☐ None

Full Name	Complete Mailing Address
N/A	

12. Tax Status (For completion by nonprofit organizations authorized to mail at nonprofit rates) (Check one)
The purpose, function, and nonprofit status of this organization and the exempt status for federal income tax purposes:
☐ Has Not Changed During Preceding 12 Months
☐ Has Changed During Preceding 12 Months (Publisher must submit explanation of change with this statement)

PS Form **3526**, August 2012 (Page 1 of 3 (Instructions Page 3)) PSN 7530-01-000-9931 **PRIVACY NOTICE**: See our Privacy policy in www.usps.com

---

13. Publication Title
Dermatologic Clinics of North America

14. Issue Date for Circulation Data Below
July 2014

15. Extent and Nature of Circulation

			Average No. Copies Each Issue During Preceding 12 Months	No. Copies of Single Issue Published Nearest to Filing Date
a.	Total Number of Copies (Net press run)		554	556
b.	Paid Circulation (By Mail and Outside the Mail)	(1) Mailed Outside-County Paid Subscriptions Stated on PS Form 3541. (Include paid distribution above nominal rate, advertiser's proof copies, and exchange copies)	206	230
		(2) Mailed In-County Paid Subscriptions Stated on PS Form 3541 (Include paid distribution above nominal rate, advertiser's proof copies, and exchange copies)		
		(3) Paid Distribution Outside the Mails Including Sales Through Dealers and Carriers, Street Vendors, Counter Sales, and Other Paid Distribution Outside USPS®	88	99
		(4) Paid Distribution by Other Classes Mailed Through the USPS (e.g. First-Class Mail®)		
c.	Total Paid Distribution (Sum of 15b (1), (2), (3), and (4))	►	294	329
d.	Free or Nominal Rate Distribution (By Mail and Outside the Mail)	(1) Free or Nominal Rate Outside-County Copies Included on PS Form 3541		
		(2) Free or Nominal Rate In-County Copies Included on PS Form 3541	73	72
		(3) Free or Nominal Rate Copies Mailed at Other Classes Through the USPS (e.g. First-Class Mail)		
		(4) Free or Nominal Rate Distribution Outside the Mail (Carriers or other means)		
e.	Total Free or Nominal Rate Distribution (Sum of 15d (1), (2), (3) and (4))	►	73	72
f.	Total Distribution (Sum of 15c and 15e)	►	367	401
g.	Copies not Distributed (See instructions to publishers #4 (page #3))	►	187	155
h.	Total (Sum of 15f and g)	►	554	556
i.	Percent Paid (15c divided by 15f times 100)	►	80.11%	82.04%

16. Total circulation includes electronic copies. Report circulation on PS Form 3526-X worksheet.

17. Publication of Statement of Ownership
If the publication is a general publication, publication of this statement is required. Will be printed in the October 2014 issue of this publication.

18. Signature and Title of Editor, Publisher, Business Manager, or Owner

Stephen R. Bushing – Inventory Distribution Coordinator

Date September 14, 2014

I certify that all information furnished on this form is true and complete. I understand that anyone who furnishes false or misleading information on this form or who omits material or information requested on the form may be subject to criminal sanctions (including fines and imprisonment) and/or civil sanctions (including civil penalties).

PS Form 3526, August 2012 (Page 2 of 3)

Printed and bound by CPI Group (UK) Ltd, Croydon, CR0 4YY

03/10/2024

01040381-0008